The Cure For Heart Disease

"Man will occasionally stumble over the truth, but usually manages to pick himself up, walk over or around it, and carry-on."

—Winston Churchill

THE CURE FOR HEART DISEASE

TRUTH WILL SAVE A NATION

Dwight Lundell, M.D.
Todd R. Nordstrom

Cover Photo: Alveraphotography.net
Interior Illustrations: Sarah Loukota
Cover/Interior Design: Judi Lynn Lake

ISBN   978-0-9790340-0-8

Printed in the United States of America

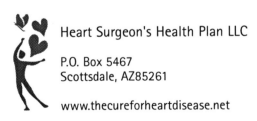

Heart Surgeon's Health Plan LLC

P.O. Box 5467
Scottsdale, AZ85261

www.thecureforheartdisease.net

To Sharon Rae Johnston, M.D.
without whose love and encouragement, my career transformation
would have been much more difficult.

To Henry and Mimi Brown,
without whose support this work would not have been possible —
better friends no man could have.

And, to Todd Nordstrom for his intelligence and the talent
to bring my accumulated knowledge, research and experience to
life on these pages in a way that will allow you to take it to Heart.

—Dr. Dwight Lundell

Table of Contents

Prologue:
A Declaration of War

Face-to-Face
with the Cure for Heart Disease

The First Meeting of the Authors

I tend to be a skeptic. That's the first thing you need to know about me.

As for Dr. Dwight Lundell, I would call him a truth seeker—he's beyond skepticism because he has the knowledge to challenge philosophy with fact. He's a guru of scientific fact.

So, how did I—the skeptic writer, known to be a tad irreverent—end up co-authoring a book with a doctor who has an unblemished reputation in cardiovascular medicine?

The first time I received a call from Dr. Dwight Lundell, asking if I would be interested in co-authoring a book with him, I admit I was extremely skeptical. The gentle, yet direct, voice on the other end of the phone politely proclaimed one of the greatest medical statements in history—heart disease had found a cure! Yes, of course I was skeptical. Was this guy actually going to say something that could change the world?

Sure, heart disease is a huge topic. But, if this doctor was going to feed me the same old mucky information that isn't making a dent in a growing heart disease epidemic, why would I care? Why would anyone care?

On that initial phone call, Dr. Lundell asked me, "Todd, how much do you know about heart disease?"

Well, I'm already a health freak. I thought I knew quite a bit. And, I thought he was about to rattle off the same information we've all heard for decades. So, it was to my surprise when he followed that initial question with, "If you do know anything about the disease, are you truly willing to change your perspective?"

Wait a second. What? Will I change my perspective? Sure, I'll change my perspective if someone would give me a reason. But, so far, no one has ever given me a real reason to change the way I think—about anything. I've written for, and about, some of the country's most recognized companies and people—billion dollar corporations, best selling authors, politicians, and high-powered executives. Plus, I have a wealth of experience writing in the health and wellness arenas—working side-by-side with leaders in medicine. Put it this way, if you can imagine it, I've probably written it at some point in my career. But, none have changed my perspective—I'm hard-headed and stubborn. So, what could Dr. Lundell possibly tell me that could truly change my perspective, change my mind, and transform my life?

That's when Dr. Lundell said something to me that I had never heard before as a writer.

"Todd, will you challenge me?" he asked. "Heart disease has found a cure."

Okay, slide the hook deep into my lip—I was intrigued. Of course, I had expected a bold statement from Dr. Lundell—anyone with his credentials surely had earned the right to plant a flag of knowl-edge—he was one of the first surgeons to operate on a beating heart. Of course he has earned the right to make a bold statement. And, without a bold statement, why would anyone want to write a book? But, why did he ask if I would challenge him?

We chatted a bit more on the phone. We set up a time to meet. And, I hung up the phone wondering if I had just bumped into something too good to be true. Can there really be a cure for heart disease?

Upon our initial face-to-face meeting, Dr. Lundell continued to sur-prise me. His demeanor is easily approachable, conversational, and even a bit laid-back—not something the average person would expect from a man who has helped shape cardiovascular medicine. He was direct, and without blinking, brilliantly recited statistical information that would ultimately bewilder the average person's thought process.

It wasn't until Dr. Lundell began speaking of his career history that I gained an insight that is rarely seen by most of us—the true mean-ing and responsibility doctors face when they take an oath. That day, I realized that medicine, at least in Dr. Lundell's perspective, was much more than a career. It was his passion and his purpose.

Somewhere in the middle of Dr. Lundell's statistical barrage about the cardiovascular epidemic our nation faces, he began reciting a story from his past—a story that quickly transformed a swarm of data into a personal mission statement. "Todd, I've saved many lives," he said. "But, as many times as I've revived life, the heartache of losing a patient never becomes a simple statistic. And, I'll be honest. As a doctor, you tend to hope that with time, you will be able to separate yourself emotionally from your patients. But, I couldn't. When your own two hands are the last chance for a person to live, and then you walk out of surgery to look a family in the eyes and tell them the bad news, it's haunting. It's horrible. And, it's especially horrible when you know that you could have saved that person's life if you had met them a few years earlier. I was walking away from a family once, hearing them mourn my horrific news—a widow and her children had just lost a husband and a father—when I realized that my thinking was backward. I knew that I had to somehow change the way I practiced medicine. We can cure heart disease. So, why don't we? That's when I knew I had to reach people before they ended up on a table in front of me. That's why I'm writing this book."

Sitting across the table from Dr. Lundell when he spoke those words made me shiver. His sincerity, passion, and even frustration were glaringly obvious. Yet, as much as I wanted to jump up and yell, "Count me in! Let's save some lives!" my skepticism took over. And, there's no doubt in my mind that he heard that skepticism in my voice when I asked, "So, you're saying that you can cure heart disease—something an entire medical community has been bumbling to cure for decades?"

He hesitated. The corner of his mouth rose slowly, smirking at my seemingly confrontational question. "This is exactly what I meant when I asked if you would challenge me," he replied. "No. I cannot cure heart disease, but you can. In fact, if we present this information correctly, anyone who reads the book will be able to save more lives than I ever could as a heart surgeon."

That's the statement that secured my intrigue and my trust. And, it's not because Dr. Lundell uses overly convincing language. In fact, as an interviewer, I would often prod Dr. Lundell for more entertaining and inspiring language. And, each time I approached a sizzling sentence, Dr. Lundell reeled me back and said, "Todd, we have the science. There's no need for sizzle."

So, you might be wondering; why am I sharing my skepticism with you before you even read the first page of Chapter 1? Well, that's a good question. I know, as a career writer, that sharing my skeptical nature isn't the best approach to promoting a theory that will revolutionize medicine. However, I think it's important to share because I believe that many of you reading this book are skeptics just like me. And, I believe it's why Dr. Lundell asked me to help him share his knowledge—to challenge him and the scientific evidence included in this book.

Throughout this book, I do challenge Dr. Lundell. Hopefully, I raise the same questions you would raise. Hopefully, I expose those raw questions that we may never get the chance to ask our family physician—much less an opportunity to ask a heart surgeon.

As you read this book, understand that Dr. Lundell wants you, like he asked of me, to challenge the material and information presented.

"When the readers of this book begin to change their lives, and fight this battle, their friends, family members, coworkers, and our culture in general will try to sabotage their newfound freedom from disease," said Dr. Lundell. "We, as a culture, need to get accustomed to challenging all information. We face this current epidemic because people didn't challenge the information they were being given. So, I want people to question this book. I want people to question everything. The facts are the only things that are real. And, with the facts, we can all win this war."

He's right. What you'll discover in this book is that the scientific facts are indisputable. You'll realize that understanding the health crisis we face isn't extremely complicated—and it can find resolve. You'll understand that there truly is a cure for heart disease. And, you'll understand that only you have the power to win this war— each and every one of you.

"This is a war," said Dr. Lundell. "It's a battle inside our bodies. It's a battle zone in our current culture. And, it's a war of information that is fought by challenging the incorrect philosophies which have made this disease a sorry epidemic—one that shouldn't exist in the first place."

Those are words that make sense. Yet, I am not a person who is easily swayed. I need direct answers. I need proof. And, I need simple solutions.

I am just like you, the reader. In the process of writing this book, I was learning the information for the first time. I was asking questions.

Now, it's your turn. The information necessary to cure heart disease is contained within the following pages. War has been declared.

— Todd Nordstrom

We are a nation under attack.
Until we come to the realization
that our current health care system is treating sickness
instead of promoting wellness, we will be plagued by epidemic.

This book is dedicated to those men and women
who refuse to lose the war against heart disease.

This book is dedicated to you.

—The Authors

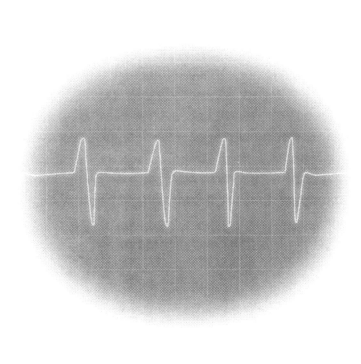

Winning the Battle and Losing the War

HEART DISEASE—THERE'S A GOOD chance it'll kill you too.

Okay, maybe this is the wrong way to start a book that focuses on heart disease. But, that opening sentence is based on statistics. And, here's the first thing you need to know about this book—it's different than all the others. That's the point.

This book will not only focus on heart disease, but on how our bodies are cellular mechanisms—connected at all levels.

Maybe you're not concerned about heart disease. Maybe you're like most people who never really buy into the terrifying statistics because, let's face it; you're healthy enough to read this book. Most of us don't think about any medical conditions until we face them ourselves. Sadly, even when we lose close family members, somehow we convince ourselves that we are different, stronger, or less likely to be afflicted.

With all the new life-saving technologies, do we really need to be concerned anyway? What about open-heart surgery—triple, quadruple, and quintuple bypass? Stellar medical technologies, like Stents and clot busting drugs, are winning more individual battles with heart disease. So, the question remaining is: why are we still losing the war?

This book is not a complicated medical journal that dives into the complexities of human physiology and disease. It's not a self-help book that gushes with inspiration. And, it's not a conspiracy theory against traditional medicine. In fact, it's quite the opposite.

This book, in its simplest form, is a transparent conversation that reveals how heart disease became an American epidemic. It's a conversation about what that epidemic looks like in our country and inside the human heart. It's a conversation with a man who has discovered a cure. And, most importantly, it's a conversation about you—your heart and your life.

What you're about to read will change your perspective—on everything you think you know about heart disease, and everything you do to prevent heart disease from this point forward.

Today begins a new chapter in your life—a new treatment of a disease that has, until this point, eluded progress. Today, everything changes—a new story is told. A war will be won!

But, haven't we heard it all before?

Hearing the same discussions for a lifetime can sound like a broken record. You don't listen to the words anymore—you simply get annoyed. Is this the case with heart disease? Have we heard the same mantra too many times? The answer is yes. And it hasn't changed anything.

Cholesterol, lifestyle habits, lack of exercise, obesity, genetics, red meat—it has all been discussed before at length. It's a tired discussion. Nothing changes. The stories don't change. The causes don't change. And the search for a cure to heart disease hasn't changed. In fact, even with all the information floating around about heart disease, its cause, and ways to prevent it, the situation has become worse—we're losing the war.

More people develop heart disease today than ever before. Every 34 seconds a person in this country dies of a heart attack—a staggering statistic considering the fact that by the time you finish reading this paragraph, another person will lose their life. And, if you're curious how many people won't live to see tomorrow—2500 people die each day of a heart attack.

All that research, all that new information, and all the fabulous technological innovations have barely made a dent. Let's be blunt, nothing changes...until now.

Imagine your life as if every step you take, every movement you make, could end or prolong someone else's life. Oops, maybe the person who is depending on you has a condition that has advanced to the point of no return—they end up with a tag around their toe, and their death was on your clock.

Or, maybe with a few slight and precise adjustments, that person could share another day with his or her family, take another long vacation, go on to live the life of their dreams, or maybe enjoy another day of simple pleasure—sipping lemonade on a park bench and watching the sun set.

Imagine it. It all depends on you. A lot of pressure? Absolutely!

Now, imagine this. What if, simply by reading this book, you could save more lives than one of our nation's best heart surgeons? Is it possible?

"Yes," says Dr. Dwight Lundell. "If everyone knew the real reasons people develop and die from heart disease, the statistics of heart disease could be dramatically reduced—and that's if they only told their family and friends."

Dr. Lundell, a heart surgeon by trade for more than twenty-five years, granted people a second chance at life every single day. Lundell specialized in coronary bypass surgery. He was the poster-child for traditional medicine. In fact, he still is. Dr. Lundell isn't airing dirty laundry about the medical establishment. He's not claiming foul by any accounts. He still supports it.

So, what makes this conversation about heart disease different?

According to Dr. Lundell, sometime during one of his 5000 or so heart surgeries amidst his quarter-century in practice, a revelation occurred—an insight into the human body that would change everything we've ever known about heart disease. It was a startling revelation that even Dr. Lundell himself couldn't ignore—a complete reversal of thought.

Lundell was saving the lives of people who needed immediate care to simply survive. What could possibly change this veteran heart surgeon's perspective?

"There I was, in the midst of surgery, looking at a patient and thinking that this man shouldn't be lying on the table," says Dr. Lundell.

"He didn't have the typical risk factors for heart disease. His choles- terol was in check. He wasn't obese. He didn't smoke. Yet, he did have one condition, the only condition that was present in each and every patient I ever saw—inflammation."

Inflammation? But, that's just a symptom or side effect—right?

The medical community has long studied inflammation as a condi- tion or a reaction to injury or infection. For decades, anti-inflamma- tory medications were prescribed without too much discussion into what it was they were actually treating other than pain. In fact, because inflammation is the number one cause of pain in the human body, anti-inflammatory medications were, and still are, typically prescribed solely to alleviate pain—from numerous conditions.

Hold on a second. Inflammation, the body's natural defense system, couldn't be causing an epidemic. It's too simple. The medical com- munity would never overlook something so obvious. Right?

What exactly is inflammation?

Inflammation is not a fancy medical term. It's exactly what you think it is—swelling, redness, heat, and pain produced in an area of the body as a reaction to injury, infection or foreign objects and substances.

Every time a mosquito stings you, a bump forms. Every time you cut your finger on a sharp object, or get burned on a hot surface, your body swells in the affected area. And, do you remember the last time you overexerted yourself—you took a long walk or jog, lifted an object that is too heavy, or even sat in an uncomfortable posi- tion for an extended period of time? The pain and soreness you feel is caused by inflammation. It's not a new discovery—it's something we all deal with every day.

So, how is inflammation related to heart disease and death?

Dr. Lundell confesses that for a long time he hadn't considered the correlation between inflammation and heart disease. Lundell, like most physicians and surgeons, simply followed standard medical protocol—wait for the patient to become ill before they are treated.

"The model is backward," says Lundell. "I had an extremely wise surgical mentor who used to say something I'll never forget. He would say that the worst thing that can happen to a patient is a diagnosis, because that's when everyone stops thinking about what is wrong. That's how the medical community treats heart disease—we wait until the situation is ready to end your life, and then open up your chest to patch the damage. It's a backward mentality."

Sadly, this was, and still is the battle cry for almost all medicine—wait for something to happen and then find a way to clean up the mess. Sure, it's a necessary approach—sick people need treatment. But, Lundell is right. If you jumped out of a tree and broke your arm, a doctor would give you a cast. And, if you went and jumped out again to break the other arm, you'd get another cast. Maybe you'd still want to jump yet another time—one more time for the sake of persistence. So, you head back to the tree to break your legs. The problem isn't breakable bones. The problem is that you jump out of trees.

If the medical community would treat the cause instead of the effect, would our country be facing an epidemic? If someone armed you with the knowledge to avoid breaking your limbs, would you listen? And, if the doctor said to you, "I can cure your problem today so that you never break another limb from falling out of tree," would you take the responsibility to help yourself avoid injury?

Can we stop jumping out of trees? And, will someone tell us to stop?

That's where this story truly begins—as a nagging suspicion that there could be more to inflammation than anyone had ever considered. Why was inflammation the only common indicator of heart disease?

What's the big deal? Anytime the body experiences an injury, inflammation is present. So what? If something goes wrong and swells, treat it. Lower the inflammation. Reduce the pain. Once the symptoms are treated, it doesn't matter what caused those symptoms. Or, does it?

"Without downplaying or criticizing the role I, or any surgeon, plays in medicine, I couldn't help thinking there was more to inflammation than suspected. What if it wasn't just a side effect? What if inflammation was in fact a culprit—the cause of cardiac arrest? If so, could I save more lives by actually treating the cause instead of simply fixing the problem? Inflammation wasn't being addressed in correlation to heart disease. Yet, the only common denominator among all the patients I've ever treated was inflammation. Why was I performing bypass surgery, when I should be curing the largest epidemic our country has ever witnessed?"

That's a good question—one that should be addressed by every doctor. However, in defense of the medical community and all the fine men and women who save lives on a daily basis, keep in mind that this question seems to escape almost every medical specialty—they all treat the symptoms instead of the cause of those symptoms. And, Dr. Lundell wasn't any different. He was in the same boat as everyone else practicing medicine. In fact, early in his career, Dr. Lundell wasn't just following standard protocol and methodology; he was helping to create it—from the day he entered medical school.

In 1967, Dr. Lundell was selected to enter the first class enrolled at the University of Arizona's brand new College of Medicine—an exciting opportunity for just 32 students, and a unique educational experience that would prove to be priceless.

"Being one of the first has its privileges," says Lundell. "We were able to form close personal and professional associations with our professors. They not only gave us the tools to become good doctors, but because we were able to form close relationships they allowed us to challenge the current philosophies. Not many students ever have that type of learning opportunity. Plus, because our group was so small, we had free roam of a beautiful new learning facility. Everything was at our fingertips."

Everything was at his fingertips. Medicine was making great strides. Technology was being introduced and tested like never before in history, and Dr. Lundell knew he could reach out and grab the steering wheel of innovation. Yet, with potential sitting in his lap, Lundell reached for the one specialty that seemed to escape progress—the human heart.

"I couldn't resist the challenge," says Lundell. "I was instantly attracted to cardiac surgery. And, maybe that's because I was introduced to the specialty by one of its brilliant pioneers, Robert M. Anderson MD. Heart disease at that time was the number one killer of people in America. Cardiac surgery was still in its infancy. Coronary artery bypass surgery was brand new and appeared to be the only available treatment for people afflicted with coronary artery disease. I knew the specialty was wide open for progress. The only question was: where would we see progress?"

Coronary bypass surgery was still brand new at the time—so new that it was only being performed on select patients. And the technology was fresh out of the box. The idea that doctors could control the circulation of a person with a heart-lung machine and restore circulation to their heart muscle with a coronary bypass to improve life inspired Lundell—it was intellectually challenging to support human life through artificial circulation. As difficult or terrifying as that may sound to those of us who may tremble facing so much pressure, Dr. Lundell says, "Pardon the pun, but that's how I fell in love with the heart. The opportunity to technologically challenge death, and quickly revive a patient to live another day fascinated me. I was hooked. I was dedicated to treating heart disease."

"I was passionate about saving lives," says Lundell. "That was my job. It was my responsibility to provide patients with a second chance. But, the thing that truly fascinated me was that each time we went into surgery we understood more. With each case we learned enough to solve a new problem and we learned why that problem existed. That's what snagged my attention—focusing on the cause of disease so we could initiate a positive change."

However, change—in any industry—takes time. In the medical community, an industry based on past philosophies and strict regulation, change is a hurdle in itself. How do you introduce new concepts that often require decades to gain approval? Change means risk.

Fortunately, change also meant insight. Change meant progress. Change was a driving force and a challenge that Dr. Lundell was compelled to face.

"Hey, if we had learned to conquer the disease at the point where it was going to take someone's life, couldn't we conquer it before they faced surgery?" asks Lundell. "That's a question I had been asking myself since my entrance into medical school. I wondered when that question would be explored, and I wanted to be part of the exploration. I had to know. And, I had to follow my instincts."

After completing his surgery residency at the University Of Arizona College Of Medicine, Dr. Lundell accepted a residency in cardiovascular surgery at Yale University. Yale's cardiac surgery department was in fact one of the pioneering centers. Yale was initiating change. Yale was changing the face of treatment. Yale was where Dr. Lundell had to be—the place with the greatest opportunity for change.

For two years Lundell studied and practiced with some of the best surgeons in the world. He spent every other night in the university's hospital caring for post-operative patients to observe and learn anything he could about their conditions.

"It was intense," he says. "We were in the operating room at least five days a week. We studied hard. We worked hard. And, we didn't get much sleep. But, we also received hours of one-on-one time with our professors learning the technical challenges you face in the operating room, and the challenges you face caring for the critically ill. The education was invaluable. There you are, face to face with brilliant surgeons—learning from the best. And, there you are, face-to-face with the patients who look to you for another day of life.

Fresh out of Yale, and ready to revolutionize the philosophies of medicine, Dr. Lundell went back to his home state of Arizona. He was on fire. He had a solution. He had a vision. He would single-handedly take on the nation's largest killer. It was great. He was great. The concept was beautiful. Dr. Lundell was going to conquer heart disease.

Would practice prove to be perfect?

For the next 25 years Lundell did what every other heart surgeon did—he saved lives. His priorities shifted from revolutionizing medicine to simply building a career to support his growing family—a lovely wife and six beautiful children.

"I was still doing what I loved," says Lundell. "And, I was helping people live another day. That's a rewarding way to make a living—emotionally and financially. I was happy. I was creating a good living to care for my family—and I had a lot of mouths to feed. Yet, I would still go to bed every night and wonder if I had lost that focus. I would struggle with the fact that I was still using mechanical solutions to treat biological problems. Quite frankly, I had become a mechanic. Don't get me wrong, fixing things when they break is a noble profession. But, I wanted more. What if things didn't have to break in the first place? What if we could conquer heart disease biologically?"

What is the biological culprit?

At the time, all the research into the biological side of heart disease was blaming cholesterol as the primary cause of heart disease. Even though Lundell wanted to take a more biological approach to treatment, he never could fully connect with the theory of cholesterol. He says the data that backed cholesterol wasn't in line with what he was seeing during surgery.

"It just didn't sit right with me," he says. "*Half of the patients that had suffered a heart attack actually had normal cholesterol. And,* when some of those patients came back for a second operation, 10 years after the first, and half of them still had normal cholesterol levels, I wondered why everyone continued to chase the theory of cholesterol. Even the nutritional studies didn't show a benefit of a low-fat, low-cholesterol diet. So there had to be something else. Something was missing."

C'mon, Dr. Lundell, everyone says that cholesterol is the killer. You'll buck the system? Everyone else is wrong?

"If a theory is wrong 50 percent of the time, why would anyone continue to believe that theory?" asks Dr. Lundell. "If I developed a new operation that only had a 50% survival rate. I would be, and should be, run out of town."

Why would the medical community believe it? Why would thousands of brilliant physicians believe it? And, what was really going on in the hearts of millions of Americans who were buying into bad advice?

The statistics of heart disease weren't getting better, they were getting worse. The medical community was mastering the art of saving lives, but why was the incidence of heart disease still growing at a terrifying, epidemic rate—the largest rate increase in history?

"We were perfecting life-saving practices while our nation, our friends, and our families faced a growing statistical probability that they would end up in our operating room," says Lundell. "I was performing by-pass like it was standard practice—bandaging the epidemic."

Bypass works. It does. It's a fantastic short-term fix. But a good comparison to the function of bypass surgery would be using duct-tape to fix a leaking pipe under your sink—it stops the leak, but it doesn't truly resolve the real issue. And, sooner or later, the real issue will arise again. What caused the pipe to leak in the first place? Was it the buildup of minerals in your water that affected the molecular strength of the pipe? Was it rust? Was it extreme water pressure and a weak spot in the pipe? Without knowing the cause of the leak, even if your commercial grade ultra hefty duct tape stands the test of the time, another leak is bound to occur because there is something wrong biologically.

"We are biological mechanisms," says Lundell. "Comparing a plumbing pipe to a human artery can work, but only if you consider the 'biology' of the pipe. One of the biggest misconceptions people make about a heart attack is that plaque clogs in the center of an artery like a pipe would clog in your sink. That's not the case. Plaque accumulates within the arterial walls—it becomes part of the artery as opposed to filling in the artery. And, that's why the discussion of inflammation is so important."

Okay, for those of us who aren't too keen on human physiology or plumbing, please excuse this graphic and somewhat disgusting comparison, which almost all of us can relate. Ready? Plaque accumulating within the wall of your artery is much like a zit growing inside your nose. Yes, it hurts to even think about. However, the zit accumulates pus inside the skin—it's part of the nasal lining. If it continues to grow, and grow, and grow, at some point it would limit your airflow in that nasal passage. At some point the zit would rupture and all the gooey stuff would shoot out into your nose and may clog the remaining space for airflow. This rupture would be similar to what happens during a heart attack, which we'll discuss in depth later in the book. The point is; a zit is inflammation—an internal swelling in the lining. It's gross. But, then again, cardiac arrest isn't pleasant to talk about either.

"I had noticed many times in the operating room that the area around the coronary artery looked inflamed like a three-day old scratch from a dirty stick," says Lundell. "All the classic signs of inflammation were there—redness, warmth, swelling and disturbed function. That's when the pieces began falling into place. If I could observe this on the outside of the artery, what was going on inside the artery? All the evidence was right there in front of me. One day it was like all the years of education, all the years spent in surgery, and all the years trying to figure out what was missing, all came down to this moment of clarity. I finally understood. And, all I had to do now was prove my theory."

Prove it, he did. He left his practice—no more patches, and no more bypasses. Lundell opened a clinic where he could test his theory on inflammation—monitoring and tracking the results of numerous patients over a period of time. And, just like he had thought, his assumptions were correct—heart disease could be biologically conquered. Inflammation was indeed the culprit.

Clinical Success Story: Debbie

A 33 year-old white female entered our clinic with the complaints of diabetes, high blood pressure, and high cholesterol. In addition, she was obese at 256 pounds. She was in rough shape—especially for her age. And, her doctor had recently told her that she needed to begin insulin injection treatments to control her diabetes, because her medications were no longer proving to be effective.

Debbie's medications included three separate pills for diabetes, two different statin drugs to lower her cholesterol, and a blood pressure lowering medication that was specifically developed for diabetic patients. Her drug costs were over $1200.00 a month.

After just 90 days in our clinic her cholesterol (LDL and HDL) and triglycerides were all normal. Her blood pressure was normal. Her blood sugar was normal—eliminating all but one diabetic medication. She had lost only 20 pounds, but she felt wonderful, was looking better and was dedicated to continue losing weight. Her medications now cost less than $100 a month. Debbie's risks of coronary disease were dramatically decreased.

And yet, there's more. Study after study and patient after patient, Dr. Lundell began to realize something he didn't expect. Reducing inflammation was not only reversing heart disease—patients who were treated at his clinic experienced other positive changes. Chronic pain was disappearing. Fatigue was diminishing. One patient who had suffered from a severe and chronic skin rash was suddenly cured. Life-long ailments vanished. Patients were feeling fantastic. Inflammation wasn't just tied to heart disease, it was tied to almost every disease and condition—Alzheimer's, stroke, diabetes, and the list continues.

But, how did all this happen? Does it make sense? Can a reduction of inflammation actually prolong your life, prevent illness and alleviate pain? And, just what exactly is Dr. Lundell's theory on inflammation?

Imagine again that you hold a human life in your hands—every move you make could determine life or death. Imagine yourself being armed with all the information necessary to understand how our nation became inflicted with a disease that can truly be conquered. Imagine you could prolong your own life, your spouse's and all your friend's and family's lives. Imagine a world without heart disease. Imagine a world where everyone gets to sip lemonade or smell flowers or go fishing without facing the thought that they could suddenly become a statistic. Imagine you have complete control. The responsibility resides solely on you.

Pressure? Absolutely!

If the life and career of Dr. Dwight Lundell can teach us anything, it's that those people who wake up everyday and believe they can change the world, actually become the people who change it.

Dr. Lundell did. Now it's your turn. Your perspective changes today. Your knowledge grows today. Your health improves today. Today you have all the tools necessary to understand what will change our nation from a dying country to a revitalized state of empowerment.

This isn't a broken record. This is a new chapter. This is the war, not the battle. This time, everything changes.

"Ironically one person, anyone who reads this book, who is armed with the right information can save more lives today than I ever could in 25 years as a heart surgeon," says Lundell. "That's power. And, it doesn't require a decade of education, or a quarter-century of experience."

Heart disease can be conquered biologically.

The answers follow. Imagine that! ⊁

Your Body, the War Zone

WARS ARE FOUGHT ON BATTLEFIELDS. Ironically, in the war against heart disease, biology (a holistic reality that our bodies are comprised of billions of interconnected cells) has dictated that one lost battle can end a war—your war.

"We all know that the human body is created from living cells—every inch of us," says Dr. Lundell. "It's not earth-shattering news to say that biology plays a role. It is the role. That being said, many doctors seem to forget this very simple fact. Humans are not machines—it's not about a body part breaking, it's about cells that are all interconnected. If there's an issue at the cellular level in one part of the body, we can safely assume that another portion could easily be affected as well."

So, that's it? That's the whole secret behind a chapter so intensely titled *Your Body, the War Zone*? Did we not know or understand that each cell in our body lives and breathes? Of course we did!

Why is biology such a big deal? Wouldn't it make sense just to talk about how we fix heart disease instead of discussing how it happens?

"Again, we cannot jump to treatment until we truly understand the cause of heart disease," says Lundell. "To understand the cause of disease, we need to understand the healthy function of the heart. Understanding biology is a 'big deal' because inflammation happens at a cellular level. It's the human body's natural defense system. It saves us, but it also can hurt us. Acute inflammation has kept our race alive for thousands of years. Think of all the viruses and infections. Think about the fevers, the cuts, bruises and slivers. Inflammation is a good thing. It's not like we can run out and get rid of it."

So, inflammation is good and bad?

Inflammation by definition means, "fire inside." It is a process by which our bodies defend us from microbes, more commonly known as germs, which try to invade us. And, before antibiotics and other modern healthcare practices were introduced, acute inflammation is what kept us alive. Kudos to inflammation for preserving our species! However, our body's natural defense system isn't always strong enough on its own—and there's good reason for that which we'll cover later in this book. Nevertheless, your body's natural defense system has the capacity to be the strongest defense army known.

Basically, our bodies were created to defend themselves. Of course, that's only if our immune systems are intact. When the body recognizes an invader like an injury, infection or toxin, a pitched battle ensues—the body wants to eliminate the invader.

Sure, it sounds a bit elementary—referring to our immune system as a stealth-fighting mechanism. However, that's precisely the case. When your body is attacked, it calls out the frontline warriors, white blood cells, by using chemical signals. And, as if they were going to war, these white blood cells receive specific instruction to defend the area of invasion.

Just like warriors, white blood cells will swarm the area of danger and secrete a variety of chemicals to defeat an infection. The chemicals are like weaponry—each designed to play a role in the battle. And, even though a comic strip description, detailing the superpowers of our body's immune system sounds intriguing and whimsical, this chapter focuses on biology. So, in the spirit of good medicine and thorough information, it is necessary to spotlight at least a portion of the science behind our natural defense systems. Biology can be tricky to comprehend, but it's not half as complicated as you might assume.

"At the core, cardiovascular biology isn't complicated at all," says Dr. Lundell. "The medical profession has complicated a very interesting conversation and insight by creating cumbersome words and terminology. The analogy of a war is very similar to our immune systems— and it offers a clearer explanation. Plus, it's more fun. And, when I've treated patients who can truly visualize what is taking place inside the arteries, inside the blood vessels, and inside the heart, those people are the ones who realize they have the power to fight the war. They can talk about what's happening. They can inform others by sharing a conversation that isn't technically boring. Those people, the ones who are informed, can talk about it and understand it enough to control it—they're empowered. It is a war. I'm simply the doctor standing by in case medical assistance is necessary. You have the power. You have the weapons to beat heart disease."

Your Body's Arsenal of Weapons: What are they?

Your body came naturally equipped with its own defense army. The chemicals secreted by white blood cells to fight invasion include oxidants, which can damage the invaders directly. Oxidation is much like rust—it's a process of breaking down the invader until it is destroyed. But, that's not the only weapon in the arsenal. The white blood cells also signal molecules such as small proteins called cytokines. Cytokines orchestrate the activities of these defensive warriors—they're the battlefield strategists.

But, if you want to know who the real warriors are—the ones that face the invasion head-on—the primary soldiers are called mono-cytes. Monocytes are an unusually aggressive type of white blood cell that are the muscle of a war—the soldiers who are deep in bat-tle, fighting invaders head-on.

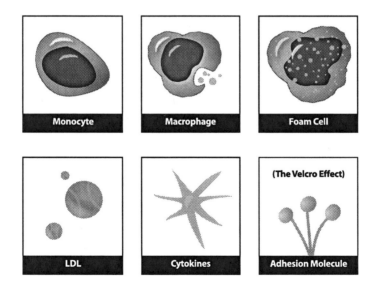

If the invader is a germ, and all the soldiers have worked together—the cytokines have orchestrated, and the monocytes have battled, some of the monocytes will graduate to the next level of aggressive behavior—converting into macrophages, which literally eat the dead and damaged germs. Weird? Yes. The thought of anything inside your body eating dead stuff seems disturbing. However, that level of uncompromised aggression exhibited by a macrophage is a good thing for your body—at least, so far.

Your body's immune system will continue to battle until every invader has been eliminated, every infection has been destroyed, and all the dead stuff has been eaten. While this fight till the death ensues, your body's warriors receive full support from their counterparts. Other cytokines are working hard to cause the small blood vessels to dilate so more blood can reach the affected area. More blood to the area of invasion means more monocytes are on their way to continue fighting, and more red blood cells are arriving carrying needed oxygen—much like a supply truck of food, medicine, and support.

This is the stage of the battle when inflammation becomes visible. The small blood vessels shift to allow the monocytes and fluid to migrate into the surrounding tissue to battle the invaders. These dilated small blood vessels actually cause the redness we see on the surface. And, other chemicals are secreted, which causes pain we feel. Pain is our signal not to use that particular part of the body while the battle continues—this is why doctors are always telling us to rest. Our doctors know that we need to allow the battle to take place. Inflammation, at this point, is serving its purpose. It's doing exactly what it was designed to do—win the battle.

We've all observed this phenomenon. And although it may seem like just a bump, or a lump, or redness, it's important to know that our bodies are fighting for our survival. One small invasion can turn into a massive ordeal if it's not confronted by inflammation. A good example would be a sliver in your finger that's not completely removed. We see the results of inflammation. The area becomes red.

It becomes swollen, it becomes warm, and it becomes painful. If inflammation didn't step in to battle infection and foreign intrusion, we could be in a serious world of hurt—the infection would spread and we would die.

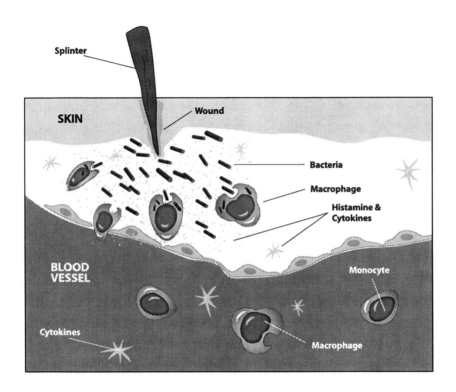

"These are the classic hallmarks of inflammation; swelling, redness, warmth, and pain," says Dr. Lundell. "This battle goes on until the invader is defeated, and then the healing process begins. The swelling will decrease, the redness will disappear, and the temperature will return to normal. Just like that, the afflicted area no longer hurts. But, if the infection becomes widespread, the symptoms will take on a new personality. We would get a fever, feel ill, and lose energy. Before antibiotics, invaders would sometimes get the upper hand—spreading like wild fire. They could overwhelm a person's army of white blood cells and eventually kill the person. So you can see that acute inflammation is necessary and beneficial. But, it can also be dangerous. Fortunately, we now have other weapons, namely antibiotics to help fight off acute infections."

Okay, so it makes sense with a sliver in the finger. But, what about heart disease?

"The sad thing about inflammation with regard to heart disease is that we can't see the lump or the redness when it's inside the body," says Dr. Lundell. "We don't know it's there. But, it's there. I've seen it in every single surgical patient I've ever treated. The process is the same, and the battle is the same—it's just in a different location."

That's the basic biology of inflammation—no matter where it occurs. To understand how inflammation causes heart disease, we now must understand the biology of a healthy heart and cardiovascular system. And, for those of us who aren't heart surgeons, this may be shocking—again, it's not really that complex.

"It's not complicated at all," says Dr. Lundell. "Many people assume that the heart is very complicated. But, if you can grasp the fact that it's only real purpose is to pump blood in and out, you're well on your way to understanding."

The human heart: 72 miracles a minute.

The average adult heart beats 72 times a minute, 100,000 times a day and 36 million times a year. During an average lifetime, the heart will pump about one million barrels of blood—enough to fill four supertankers. Basically, it's a workhorse. Each time the heart beats it circulates blood through a huge network of vessels, arteries, veins, and capillaries. In fact, the network is so vast that if you stretched out your blood vessels along side the road they would extend for 60,000 miles. That's like driving from Los Angeles to New York City, cross-country, almost 22 times!

"There was a time when the heart was thought to be a pump connected to static pipes, like the plumbing in your house," says Dr. Lundell. "It is more than that, but it's still not that complicated. We now know that the cardiovascular system is indeed a system with two separate circulation networks. The right side of your heart pumps blood to the lungs where it eliminates carbon dioxide and takes in oxygen."

That's simple enough—carbon dioxide out, oxygen in. All our cells need oxygen to survive. And, we have 60,000 miles of blood vessels to carry oxygen and nutrients to those cells.

"The left side of the heart pumps blood to our body to deliver nourishment and eliminate waste," says Lundell. "Each side has a role to play. One side pumps to make the blood usable to the cells and the other side distributes it to the cells."

So far, it's not complicated at all. In fact, Dr. Lundell says that the heart just may be the "dumbest" part of the entire human cardiovascular system.

"In spite of all the characteristics we associate with a heart, it has the least control over what happens in our cardiovascular system. The amazing thing about our cardiovascular system is its ability to monitor the body and change the circulation to accommodate different situations. Whether you are running, lying down, under stress or exposed to extreme temperatures, your cardiovascular system is constantly monitoring and making the necessary changes for your survival. It's a brilliant system—but none of the monitoring takes place in the heart."

That's interesting. And, it may be the first real indicator that the human body isn't just a machine made up of singular parts, operating on their own. Imagine for just one second that even one inch of the 60,000 miles of blood vessels senses a problem. How does that one small problem affect the rest of the mileage? Let's say you planned to take the trip from L.A. to New York, and you were going to drive the distance between the two cities 22 times. What if you're car overheated on the first trip? Wouldn't it be nice to have a team of analysts following your commute and monitoring all your systems? This is how the vessels monitor blood flow—adapting and adjusting at each mile of the trip. Smart blood vessels? Yes. Brilliant.

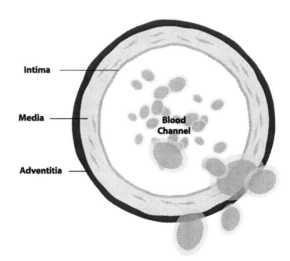

"Each of our arteries is composed of three distinct layers," says Lundell. "The inside layer is thin. It's called the endothelium. The

second layer is called the medial layer. It's composed of smooth muscle cells, which allows the blood vessels to expand or contract—increasing or decreasing blood flow to a particular organ or tissue as needed. And, the outer layer is called the adventitia. It's the casing layer that separates the blood vessels from all the other tissues. All layers serve a distinct purpose in the monitoring and adaptation process to regulate blood flow."

How do these layers know what to do and when to do it?

"Blood flow through our arteries is carefully controlled by a nervous system, along with certain hormones and chemicals," says Dr. Lundell. "The nervous system sends signals to tell the cardiovascular system how it should react. And, the nervous system receives signals from the cardiovascular system as well. For example, when you exercise, your heart can pump twice as fast and circulate four times as much blood as it can while you rest. Basically, your muscles need more oxygen so the vessels adapt the blood flow. In cold temperatures, arteries in the skin constrict to conserve body heat and protect vital organs. Again, the vessels are reacting to stimuli and adapting. And, even on smaller levels, if we get embarrassed, the blood vessels in our face dilate, making us feel warm and look red. All these responses are controlled and initiated by a complete system of monitoring. Yes, there are a lot of signals being sent and received constantly. But, no matter how much is going on in your body, it's the same basic concept. And, it's not that complicated when you remove all the medical terminology from the discussion."

Still, fairly simple, right? Basically, there's one single process that regulates blood flow to various parts of the body to achieve a different goal—like preserving heat, providing more oxygen, or protecting vital organs. It is simple. But, with all these signals being transferred back and forth at the same time, how does the cardio-vascular system know what to do first? Is it first come, first serve? Or is there preference?

"Of course there's preference," says Lundell. "We wouldn't last too long if the cardiovascular system didn't have a preference. The cardiovascular system protects the crucial organs first. The brain gets about 20% of the blood supply, the kidneys receive 20%, and no matter what the scenario, the heart gets at least 5%—it protects itself. That's standard. However, if there's trauma to the body, like blood loss or shock, blood is diverted away from other tissues and organs to protect these vital organs."

That's good news for those of us still jumping out of trees. If we lose a leg, our vital organs receive the most blood, and our face won't turn red from embarrassment.

"An example that we could see on a daily basis would be something as simple as exercise. Let's say you go for a bike ride. During your ride, blood vessels in the muscles will dilate providing more blood flow to the muscles. While that's happening, blood vessels in the stomach will contract to reduce the blood flow. The blood is flowing to the area where it is needed most."

Imagine that. The blood vessels really are the "brains" behind the cardiovascular system—dilating or contracting as needed. The vessels, not the heart, send blood preferentially to one place or another, controlling numerous bodily functions. The heart actually has the least control. And, while your heart rate can change due to different stimuli, the amount of blood that is pumped is actually controlled by how much blood is delivered by the rest of the cardiovascular system.

"Our cardiovascular system is amazing," says Lundell. "It is a coordinated, synchronized system that allows us to go about our activities without concerns. It's beautiful. It's simple. It's precise. It's perfect. Unless, of course, it's unhealthy."

Unhealthy? Uh-oh. Yes, that is the reason that we're having this conversation. It's the reason we're having a discussion about biology, and the interconnected systems. It is the reason that Dr. Lundell saw a better way to treat heart disease. And, it's the reason for every reader of this book to realize that they too were provided with a system that can operate without fail. Sadly, the perfect system is unhealthy in more Americans today than ever before in history.

What makes the perfect system fail?

In a healthy cardiovascular system, blood vessels have a very smooth lining, they're elastic, and can dilate and constrict in response to stimuli as needed. So, what happens to make the system unhealthy? How do we get from this beautiful vascular system to a situation where the arteries are hard as rocks—jammed full of yellow, squishy, margarine-looking material that limits blood flow, creates clots and eventually gives us a heart attack or stroke?

What happens?

Inflammation happens. The same inflammation that saves our life can also kill us. Remember, we're discussing biology. Everything is connected. And so is this discussion. This is where all those tricky medical words you learned earlier come back to make sense.

"Normally, the inner layer of the artery is very smooth," says Dr. Lundell. "It's made up of a single layer of endothelial cells. However, in the presence of some of the chemicals associated with inflammation (like cytokines), the lining of the blood vessel can become more like Velcro—acting like an adhesive and grabbing on to the circulating monocytes (remember those warriors that fight infections?). The now sticky, adhesive lining grabs onto the monocytes, making them think that there is a battle to be fought."

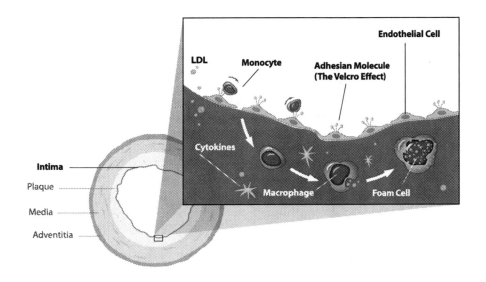

This is the beginning of inflammation gone bad.

Can you control it? How do you control it? And, if your body is simply reacting, how do you change a natural physiological process?

"This is biology," says Dr. Lundell. "The beautiful thing about biology is that it doesn't take a heart surgeon to change it. In fact, every person reading this book has the power to change biology. All the tools are there for your body to prevent heart disease without drastic measures. They've been there all along. But, this isn't just a biological problem within our bodies. It's a biological problem within our culture and the way we've perceived a disease—a disease that has turned into an epidemic."

Biology of culture? Is it a possibility that our culture, the messages, and the medicine are also interconnected? Has the biology of our culture created an epidemic?

What really happens when inflammation goes bad? What does it look like? And, could inflammation end your life?

"Everyone has the scars of inflammation," says Lundell. "If everyone is at risk, the real question is; what can we do about it? And, are we ready to face the biology of a heart attack?" ⌘

three

The Good and The Bad Turn Ugly

SO FAR WE'VE USED A lot of ugly descriptions. And, maybe the mere focus on biology and blood makes you a bit queasy. Understandably, biology can be cumbersome to comprehend, the discussion of blood can be a tad graphic, and the simple fact that you know this conversation will soon turn to demise can seem bleak. Cardiovascular malfunction can be a dismal discussion. However, consider the horrific truth if we avoid this discussion—disease, death and continued epidemic?

This is where we face the ugly truth.

"A lot of people don't like to talk about disease," says Dr. Lundell. "I think it's more than just an adversity to the biological grossness—the blood and the guts of disease. For many of us, a discussion about a diseases that the medical community has failed to overcome, simply makes us feel vulnerable—a feeling that we don't understand disease, and even if we did, we wouldn't have any control over it."

Is that the case? Are we, the regular people of the world who don't have degrees in medicine, frightened to face disease?

Disease is ugly. For anyone who has ever had the nauseating privilege of dissecting an animal or even a human cadaver in a high school or college classroom, knows that our internal organs aren't necessarily pretty. And, if you've ever seen a diseased organ up-close, it's gruesome enough to change your lifestyle on the spot. A cancerous human lung in your hands can make a 3-pack-a-day smoker quit instantaneously. But, it doesn't stop there. The internal anatomy of any species, especially if it's unhealthy, can initiate years of healthy living. Try dissecting an obese cat. French fries will no longer be a staple in your diet. That's a guarantee—even though a cat doesn't make stops at a drive-through.

One glimpse at biology gone bad and you'll be a changed person.

"We don't have the luxury of truly showing people the progression of the epidemic we face," says Dr. Lundell. "I've seen it. I've held it in my hands. It's not pretty. However, those who can understand this discussion—and realize they are equipped with the same physiology as every one else—hold the power to change what is happening in their body. This discussion might be gross. But, it's the gross discussion that will lead to a beautiful outcome. We can reverse the ugly stuff. It's that simple."

So, bear with us for another discussion in biology. And, be prepared. If you thought the old way of thinking about a heart attack was gross, this conversation will really turn your stomach.

For decades it was thought that heart attacks happened when a bunch of fatty gunk clogged in your arteries—the blood would just get plugged behind the gunk and you would die. That's not the case. The reality is actually much worse.

"The gunk is still there," says Lundell. "But, now we know that a heart attack is much more complicated. People don't die because of the gunk. They die when the plaque ruptures and the fatty, toxic gunk spills into the artery and a blood clot forms to stop the blood flow."

Go ahead, imagine it, and feel free to vocalize,"Eeew!" That rupture or explosion in your arteries could happen at any given second—whether or not you have any of the typical risk factors—heredity, obesity, poor diet, lack of exercise, high cholesterol or even smoking. Rupture is due to inflammation—plain and simple.

Heart attacks happen quickly. Heart disease takes time.

"There's one good thing about a heart attack that everyone should know," says Lundell. "If we all reframe the concept of a heart attack, and realize that it starts with heart disease, we can begin to backtrack. We can understand that no one dies instantly—it's a process. If heart disease can progress, then surely it can regress. Right? And, that's where we find power."

Okay, so you're ready to see the ugly disease. We explained the healthy cardiovascular system. We explained the biology of inflammation. And now, you'll see the diseased cardiovascular system, and how inflammation can cause that sudden burst—the moment we like to call "cardiac arrest."

No, we don't have the luxury of handing you a diseased heart to accompany this book. But, through explanation and your awareness of the heart that is beating inside your chest, you'll be armed with some very straightforward knowledge that could save your life. So, hang on through this discussion, no matter how nasty it gets. You'll discover what's actually happening inside your body. And, once you understand this, the information will empower you to control the disease, help others avoid it, and help you understand how we all can change a culture that has relentlessly promoted the downfall of the human heart.

Okay, so let's imagine that you eat a meal. Sometimes you eat really healthy meals and sometimes, well, not so healthy. All types of foods contain things our bodies use and don't use. And, our body is pretty good at handling all types of foods—even cholesterol, which has been deemed the 'evil culprit'.

"The reason cholesterol has been blamed for so long is because it's at the forefront of the discussion," says Dr. Lundell. "We know that certain foods contain cholesterol. And, our bodies manufacture cholesterol. We actually need cholesterol. It's not the substance that is killing millions of Americans."

Wait. Why are we starting our evil and ugly discussion with cholesterol when it's not really the culprit?

Cholesterol is not evil.

Cholesterol is, in fact, vital to human life. Up to 50% of all cell walls are made up of cholesterol. Cholesterol is the precursor to many critical compounds and hormones including male and female sex hormones, vitamin D and bile acids.

"Approximately 80% of cholesterol is manufactured in the body," says Dr. Lundell. "Almost all cells can make cholesterol. But the majority is synthesized in the liver. Healthy people maintain a relatively constant blood cholesterol level no matter how much cholesterol they eat. If we consume more cholesterol through dietary sources, then our liver makes less cholesterol to even it out. The synthesis of cholesterol is controlled mostly by insulin. The pancreas produces insulin as a response to ingested sugars and starches—to control blood sugar levels. High levels of insulin, resulting from high intake of sugars and starches, stimulate the production of cholesterol and disrupt the normal control (or balancing) mechanisms of the body."

"In our clinic," he continues, "the reduction of blood cholesterol, when we reduced consumption of sugars and starches, was dramatic. The patients who followed the diet and took their supplements had their cholesterol and triglyceride levels return to normal. With many of these patients we were able to discontinue both high cholesterol and diabetic medications."

Clinical Success Story: Maggie

A 65 year-old white female entered our clinic with high blood pressure and high cholesterol. She was taking a statin for her cholesterol and two medications for high blood pressure.

At the end of 90 days, Maggie's weight had dropped from 167 lbs. to 135. Her cholesterol had dropped from 240 to 138. Her triglycerides had dropped from 210 to 85 Her LDL had dropped from 130 to 81. And, her blood pressure had dropped from 144/84 (with medication) to 122/66 (with no medication). Maggie's results were astonishing. Her health was in a fragile state before she entered the clinic.

Clinical Success Story: Jack

A 67-year-old man with known coronary artery disease, high blood pressure, and high cholesterol entered our clinic. Within 30 days he had lost a total of 20 pounds. His blood pressure, which was 162/82 on medication, dropped to 114/66 without medication. His cholesterol and LDL returned back to healthy levels. Most important-ly, Jack's C - reactive protein, which was 5.1 (dangerous-ly high) when he entered the clinic, dropped to just 1.4 — a much more acceptable level. Jack was lucky that he changed his life. I don't think he would have survived very long otherwise.

So, cholesterol is necessary? And, it's not unhealthy?

"It is necessary," says Dr. Lundell. "Low-density lipoprotein (LDL) carries cholesterol to the tissues for all types of biologic processes—most of which are healthy. Under normal circumstances, cholesterol passes in and out of the blood vessel wall without difficulty. Our bodies actually use cholesterol for a number of biological processes. But, low-density cholesterol, or LDL cholesterol, is what the medical profession has deemed the 'bad cholesterol.' That's the cholesterol we've seen on TV, read about in magazines and heard about on the radio from talk-show doctors. The fact is; it really isn't bad at all. It's simply a carrier of cholesterol from the liver, where it is synthesized, manufactured, and distributed to the tissues to be used. However in the presence of high blood sugar or from oxidative stress, the LDL experiences chemical changes and the body interprets it as dangerous."

Danger? Okay, remember when we talked about those instances where our bodies perceive danger due to trauma or infection?

Remember the Velcro Effect that happens when certain chemicals are released by our little warriors that step in to fight off the danger? Well, here we are, right back at the sticky stage. Your body senses danger and all those little Velcro-like feelers pop out due to the presence of weird chemicals. The Velcro pops out, the immune system warriors attach, and your body declares war.

This is a heated battle. The monocytes convert to macrophages. The macrophages, being the aggressively gross, "I'll eat the dead or foreign garbage in my body" warriors, consume the LDL to eliminate the perceived invader—they eat it to remove it. They gobble up every last drop.

"If the macrophages consume enough oxidized LDL cholesterol, they can actually choke on it and die," says Dr. Lundell. "Remember, they're living cells too. And, they will fight and consume until the invader is completely gone."

So, they eat, and eat, and eat. And, they grow in size just like any living organism would if it continued to eat. They get plump. They get fat. They keep consuming and when they reach a certain point, they take on the appearance of foam—which pathologists have adequately named "foam cells."

"If the inflammatory stimuli are not stopped, and if the macrophages continue to eat until they choke and die, they release toxins of their own into the arterial wall," says Dr. Lundell. "We can see this in surgery as a yellow streak inside the artery wall. This is called the 'fatty streak.' And, it is the beginning of significant heart disease."

Again, feel free to vocalize your disgust. "Eeew. Foam."

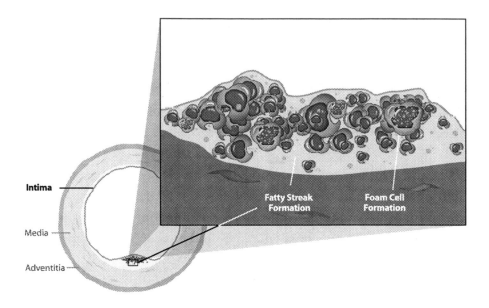

Intima

Media

Adventitia

Fatty Streak Formation

Foam Cell Formation

Unfortunately, most Americans harbor these fatty streaks beginning as early as teenage years. And, once you have a fatty streak, the danger of heart disease is present. That's a scary thought. Many of us have harbored a fatty streak since our own high-school biology class when we were getting grossed out by dead frogs. We had the foam at a young age. Our bodies were in danger all along.

Danger strikes at a young age.

It's hard to grasp—danger at a young age. However, the danger makes perfect sense. Consider this. When the body attempts to build a wall to contain the fatty streak, like scaring, our immune systems sense more danger and send even more warriors to the battle. Yikes. The warriors then try to break down the scar tissue. This creates a cyclical battle inside your body. More scarring means increased troops on your front lines. The cycle will continue if it's not interrupted. And, over time, if your body's defense system is successful, it will weaken the arterial wall, chewing through the scar tissue, to allow a rupture—pop!

A continuous cycle of the inflammation process—how long does it take to kill you?

"If the inflammation cycle continues, this fatty streak will continue to grow into what is known as a plaque—basically a larger accumulation of foam cells," says Dr. Lundell. "Some of these foam cells die and release the accumulated lipids. This can develop into what's known as the lipid core—a soft, yellow liquid substance that resembles margarine."

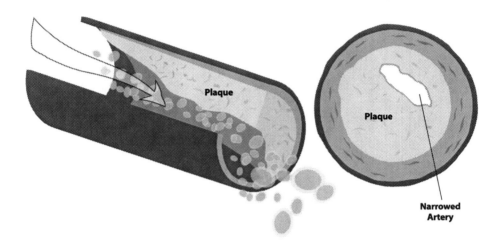

Great. That's a lovely thought—guts of dead cells that look like butter spewed throughout your arterial walls and expanding without permission. That's gross. It sounds like it happens so quickly—without warning, or any way of stopping the process. And, if it begins when most of us are teenagers, how can we still be walking around today?

"At this point, if the inflammation is stopped, the artery will heal the affected portion with what is called a fibrous cap," says Lundell. "This just goes to show how perfect our bodies are at compensating. Our bodies will do numerous things to protect us. A fibrous cap is made up of fibrous scar tissue. It remains stable in the absence of a new inflammation. Cardiologists call this process, 'a stable plaque.' This means that it is not dangerous unless it's big enough to compromise blood flow in the coronary artery. Thankfully, this is why most of us are still alive today—the inflammation process was interrupted."

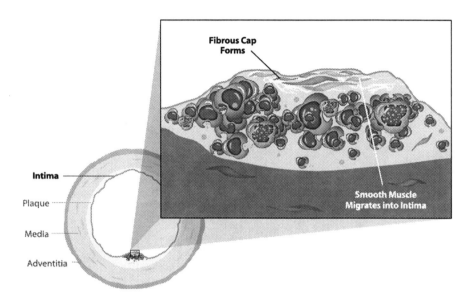

So, basically, our bodies are continually trying to protect us. And, over a life-span, depending on how we treat our bodies and our own genetic individuality, this process just proves that heart disease isn't instantaneous. It's a slow progression.

"Anyone can see that if you interrupt this process at any given point, by reducing inflammation, the process can stop," says Lundell. "But, if we don't interrupt it, the inflammatory condition will continue until it kills us—consistently accumulating more foam cells. More foam cells mean more macrophages. They will continue to eat until they die. The lipid core continues to expand. More chemicals are released, which weaken and destroy the fibrous cap.

And the inflammation cycle will elevate with time."

Of course it will elevate—the bigger the perceived battle, the more warriors that will be sent to war.

When does it turn into a heart attack?

"Inflammation, your body's own defense system, will kill you," says Dr. Lundell. "If the fibrous cap ruptures, the soft lipid gunk is pushed into the bloodstream. It's much like popping a boil. Pop, out it goes into your bloodstream. The blood recognizes the gunk as a foreign substance. When the blood recognizes a foreign substance, a blood clot is immediately formed to prevent the gunk from spreading."

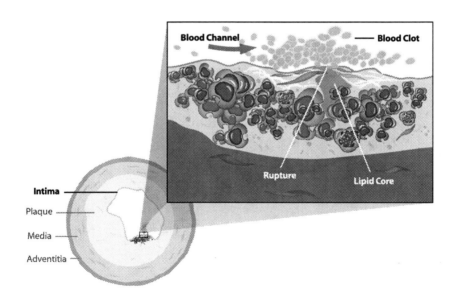

Again, our bodies are at work protecting us. However, an instant blood clot, instantly blocks blood flow, which deprives the heart muscle of any oxygen. Without oxygen, the tissue begins to die.

Tissue death is basically a dying of cells—they need oxygen to survive. And, when that tissue is the heart muscle, it's called a heart attack.

"A little anatomy lesson here would be helpful," says Dr. Lundell. "There are two blood vessels that supply the heart muscle with blood—the right coronary and the left coronary. The left coronary is divided into the left anterior descending, and the circumflex artery. If the left main artery closes suddenly, we die. If the left anterior descending closes, the risk of sudden death is very high. Closure of the right coronary artery, or the circumflex branch, typically do not result in sudden death. Nevertheless, all closures are bad. Unless a heart attack is interrupted by clot busting drugs, death of the heart muscle occurs. Dead heart muscle turns to scar tissue. Scar tissue does not function normally as heart muscle. Scarring causes the heart to pump less efficiently. And, if enough scarring occurs, congestive heart failure is the result."

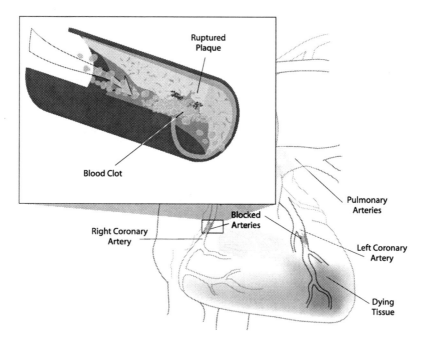

Well, that's something most of us didn't know. There is a difference between heart attack and heart failure. Heart attacks can go virtually unnoticed. We could be walking around and not have a clue. That's a scary thought considering that the cycle of inflammation would most likely be in the midst of heated battle beyond our imagination—building on momentum to cause sudden death.

"A heart attack can go unnoticed," says Lundell. "That doesn't mean it will go unnoticed. Most people feel a heart attack—it may be the last thing they feel. But, a person who experiences heart failure, well, they'll know it without question. It doesn't feel good."

The symptoms of heart failure are shortness of breath and swelling of the legs among other things. And, just so none of us feel too confident because we don't feel any symptoms, Dr. Lundell says, "The thing that's hard to predict is the size and degree of tissue death. If a heart attack occurs in a specific area, or is large enough, sudden death is the result. You won't have any warning. You're done."

So, why is a heart attack the first sign or symptom of heart disease for so many people?

If unstable plaque ruptures and was not big enough to diminish blood flow and cause symptoms, a person may never know anything happened," says Dr. Lundell. "This is why heart attacks catch so many people off guard. They could have accelerated heart disease and never feel a thing. As a matter of fact, 80% of all heart attacks occur from ruptured plaque."

That doesn't mean that tissue death has occurred. If you have a heart attack and get to a hospital soon enough, doctors will give you a clot-dissolving drug.

"These drugs restore blood flow by dissolving the clot," says Lundell. "Notice I said that they dissolve the clot. They don't dissolve plaque. This is very important to clarify. The blood clot, not the cholesterol, caused the acute heart attack."

So, in the end, it's not cholesterol. In fact, cholesterol had little to do with the heart attack. Consider it the vehicle that drives you out to our evil tree that we discussed earlier. Normally, you'd pass by the tree. But, sometimes the vehicle stops, simply because the conditions for jumping are perfect. And, that's when the battle ensues. Just because you're near the tree, and the conditions for jumping—sunny skies, light cumulous clouds, and few chirping birds—are perfect, doesn't mean you jump. But, if the tree wins the battle, calls you over to its branches, you could end up breaking something. And, it's not going to be pretty.

How do we interrupt the cycle of inflammation? What creates the perfect conditions for our bodies to allow the process to kill us? And, how did cholesterol get such a bad reputation in the world of heart disease? These are all great questions. And, you guessed it, the answers will soon follow.

However, by now you're probably sick and tired of reading about biology. You're probably asking yourself a million questions. And, you may feel a little overwhelmed because, let's face it, lowering your cholesterol is easy—stop eating shrimp and steak. Lowering your fat consumption is easy—stop eating fried foods. But, if your own natural defense system is causing your demise, how do you control it?

Is everything you've learned about staying healthy a bunch of bunk?

"Everything we've known about controlling heart disease, and many diseases for that matter, is simply incorrect," says Dr. Lundell. "That doesn't mean that all of it is wrong. But, the focus is wrong. It's way off-course. And, people have been mislead for the wrong reasons. How did a nation, a culture, and a medical community take such a wrong turn? People will be shocked to know the truth."

What is the truth?

"I've had people ask me how much healthier they'll be if they take control of their heart health," says Dr. Lundell. "I always respond by reverting to the facts—the science proves everything. I didn't invent biology. I didn't invent inflammation. The secrets have always been there for us to reveal. And, the changes a person can make in their own life are dramatic if they choose to take control today. That said, it is my strong belief that if we control inflammation, we would age much more slowly, feel fantastic, and function better—today and well into our later years of life."

What does typical aging look like inside our arteries?

"A picture tells a thousand words," says Lundell. "If you see the difference between typical aging and unhealthy aging, it's enough to stop you in your tracks.

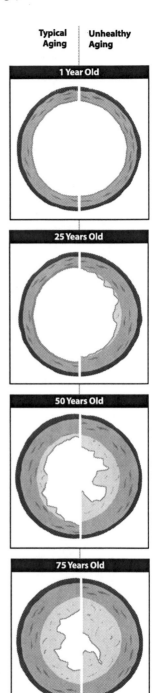

Typical Aging | Unhealthy Aging

1 Year Old

25 Years Old

50 Years Old

75 Years Old

However, I'd like to take this one step further. I will take the bold step forward and challenge even what the medical establishment refers to as "typical" aging. In my opinion, "typical" doesn't even come close to the potential we all have to save our own lives."

What's possible? Dr. Lundell probably said it best. A picture is worth a thousand words.

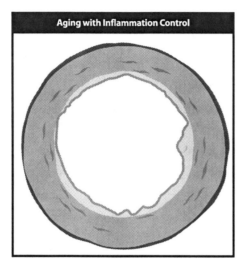

Ready to take control? ✕

Smack Dab in the Middle
of an Epidemic

HOW'D WE END UP FIGHTING for our lives?

Medical technology is much like any household piece of electronic equipment—it's outdated before it ever makes it to market. The only difference between a personal computer and a piece of medical technology is that the medical technology undergoes years of time consuming and rigorous testing before it can be released to the public.

So, you'd think that with medical technology advancing at such an aggressive pace, standard thought and practice would advance as quickly—even if it had to wait through a decade of testing. Sadly, it doesn't.

Why hasn't it advanced? Why are we still treating diseases only after they infringe on a person's life? Why are we still waiting for patients to become sick before problems are addressed?

Here's the biggest spoiler to that list of questions. The information contained in this book isn't new—it's been around for a long time. So why isn't anything changing?

What? Wait a minute.

This isn't a new theory?

If you're reading this book and thinking that Dr. Lundell is the first surgeon to challenge the standard system and methodology in the medical community, you'd be mistaken. In fact, discussions similar to the one presented in this book have been going on for centuries.

Thomas Henry Huxley, one of the most notable intellectual giants of the 19th century, a pioneering genius whose influence was felt throughout science, education, politics, and medicine, probably best summarized the same conversation we're discussing today when he wrote; *The great tragedy of science is the slaying of a beautiful hypothesis by an ugly fact.*

He's right. If the facts don't support a theory, especially when we're fighting an epidemic and people are dropping like flies around us, why would we continue to chase that theory?

No, the theories in this book aren't new. The system and thought to treating heart disease has been challenged numerous times. So, why is Dr. Lundell's approach different?

"I said it before and I'll continue to repeat it," says Dr. Lundell. "If a theory is wrong more than half the time, it really doesn't deserve continued discussion. Cholesterol shouldn't be a discussion. So, why am I going to talk about it? If all the messages we receive from the medical establishment, the government, and from pharmaceutical companies are missing a critical element and misleading the American people, it has to be faced—head on. Today, the cholesterol theory is so prevalent in the public. And because we're all bombarded on a daily basis with print and television ads for cholesterol lowering medications, we must deal with it. That's why we're talking about it. And, today, we can finally provide both the history of the heart disease epidemic and the solution—the facts support the cause and the cure."

Those facts had to come from somewhere. And, if they've been around for so long, how in the world did we end up in such a sad state of heart health?

Well, just take a walk down memory lane and it's obvious to see that public perception has always clashed with the facts. Imagine how many times Christopher Columbus was challenged when he presented a theory that the world wasn't flat. The science, at least as much as they had at the time, was there to support his claim, but public perception had always dared the nay-sayers to actually sail to the edge—fearing the possibility of taking a nose dive into a great abyss.

These types of stories beg us to ask, why don't we simply trust the science? How does a public perception that is not supported by fact become an ongoing mantra? And, because these magically mythical public perceptions aren't supported by scientific facts, how dangerous are they to the public who buy into the theories?

Again, the typical discussion about heart disease has become tired. It's been a medical headliner for as long as most of us can remember. The discussion has been beaten to death—death in epidemic proportions.

"It's not like someone sat down and decided to create a bad rumor," says Dr. Lundell. "All the things we thought we knew about heart disease arose for a reason. Yet, most people would be surprised by those reasons. Most of the information we've received has no scientific foundation whatsoever. And that's a sad statement."

A prescription without scientific support?

Huh? Did he say that most of the information we receive about heart disease isn't based on scientific findings?

Uh-oh. He did.

Everything you thought you knew about health is about to change—right now. Your world is about to become round. No more fear of taking a nosedive from misleading information.

Heart disease has been around forever. However, the prevalence of the disease emerged when humans converted to an agricultural based society from a hunting and gathering society. That's when the medical community saw the first real glimpse of the disease, even though it was still very rare.

And, even though most people would assume that a richer, more industrialized and technologically advanced society would be a healthier society, the statistics prove otherwise. Basically, as the wealthiest nation in the world, we've dropped our spears and became a bunch of "fat-cats."

Obviously, health care got better. Doctors learned to fix more ailments and save more lives. But our people—the same ones revolutionizing world technology—were accumulating disease like it was a new fashion statement. There was no more hunting. There was no more gathering. There was just a bunch of sick people dying from heart attacks. And, the richer, more civilized our country became, the more our hearts suffered.

Is that progress?

Imagine if your personal computer kept advancing with new ways to mend unwanted technical glitches, but the more you fixed the glitches the worse the real problems grew. Would you question how to find better fixes for the glitches? Or, would you figure out why there were glitches in the first place?

Concern about heart disease didn't really arise until the aftermath of World War II. All of a sudden, men began to die of heart attacks—these men had supposedly been considered healthy, strapping men. The whole concept of heart disease was an entirely new phenomenon. And, not too many years after that, autopsies of soldiers killed in the Korean War began to reveal more startling facts. "The typical soldier in the Korean War was 22 years old," says Dr. Lundell. "Suddenly, these young men were coming back in body bags and 77% of them were showing evidence of coronary artery disease. The disease ranged from simple fatty streaks to significant plaque formation. So, what was going on?"

Remember, danger can strike at a very young age. But, this was startling—it shocked the American public, the medical establishment and the U.S. Government. Why was this happening? These dead soldiers were just kids.

What happened when these statistics were released to the public? Well, everybody freaked out. That's what happened.

The results of these findings basically threw the government and the medical community into high alert. The whole concept of heart disease was still brand new. Overnight, it became a disease that could strike anyone at any age.

Panic! Run for your lives. Heart disease is coming to get you!

All the scurrying, and all the panic, combined with the desperate cries from the public, resulted in the most well-known medical study on heart disease to date. The Framingham Study began in 1948. It followed more than 5000 healthy men and women and basically sought a common physiological indicator of those who would be stricken with heart disease.

Whew! Wipe your brow—we're all saved. Finally someone is studying heart disease. But, would the new study uncover the truth?

"You can't really blame or place judgment on the early Framingham Study," says Dr. Lundell. "Realize that this was really the first comprehensive study of its kind, and they were starting with an open slate. They were simply looking for a common thread that linked heart disease to something—something they could say grouped people together or increased their risk of developing the disease. And, their findings set the standard for what the medical community is still chasing today—the good findings, and the bad."

Yikes. Take a deep breath. The Framingham Study began in 1948. Consider all the medical advancements that have taken place over the last 60 some years—since that study launched. We're still chasing the same theories? Early on, the researchers in the Framingham study weren't even sure what they were looking to discover about heart disease.

Here's a funny thought. Imagine if Christopher Columbus, or any explorer for that matter, had never set sail to actually prove that the world was round. Let's say no one had ever discovered the western world. The British would still be in Europe today creating technology—satellites and high-tech equipment to measure all kinds of scientific stuff—without ever considering this huge chunk of land on the other side of the ocean. At least now they can blame the depletion of the ozone on the American obsession for hairspray.

It's comical to consider. But, it raises a great question. How accurate can science be if no one is willing to wander out and discover the whole truth?

So, was the early Framingham Study bad?

"The Framingham Study quickly discovered a few things that have been important in the fight against heart disease—like the fact that cigarette smoking increases a person's odds for heart disease," says Lundell. "They also quickly discovered that some heart attacks happened without any symptoms—the silent and painless heart attack I mentioned earlier. And then, in 1961, the study discovered cholesterol. This is when everybody kind of lost track. Instead of looking for all variables that could contribute to heart disease, their focus became narrow."

It's important to note that the Framingham Study continued following the lives of the initial participants and two subsequent generations to track and monitor the onset of heart disease. And, it's also important to note that the study has continued to build a wealth of knowledge that has been extremely useful in the fight against heart disease. Yet, everyone still took the findings on cholesterol and went to town.

So, isn't that science? It's definitely a study of a large group of people. And, it revealed a ton of great things about a nasty disease. Can't we just be happy with finding gobs of cholesterol?

"The question goes back to what we already discussed," says Lundell. "Maybe the study found that high cholesterol levels were prevalent. But, what did that cholesterol mean? What else was different in those people who developed heart disease? What does cholesterol do inside the body?"

Yea, what did it mean? Of course, anyone reading this book already knows what cholesterol does inside the body from reading the last chapter. Dietary cholesterol, the cholesterol we eat, means very little. Still, scientists continue to chase it today. At least they should get points for persistence, eh?

"When the medical community finds something like cholesterol, it runs with it," says Dr. Lundell. "And, we need to give credit to those who instantly searched for a way to reduce cholesterol. That was taking the bull by the horns—even though it was the wrong bull."

How could anyone deny that so many (okay, well at least half) of the people in the Framingham Study who developed heart disease had high cholesterol? Half of the study group isn't a big number. However, it was something for the medical community and the public to grab onto—a valiant fight to cure an epidemic. So, the Framingham Study was released. From that day forward, high levels of cholesterol were associated with increased chances of heart attack in middle-aged men. But not for women.

Not for women? Well, what the heck, let's chase it anyway. Doesn't that seem silly? You would think it they would consider the lack of evidence in women. But, they didn't. They chased it anyway. Medicine continued to knock at the cholesterol door saying, "reduce it no matter what"—but never questioning how it affected the body.

"At first they blamed our diets," says Dr. Lundell. "That seemed rational. How do most things get inside our bodies? They said the consumption of fat caused elevated blood cholesterol. If that was the case, then we'd be in great shape. Fat consumption is easy to track and monitor."

Uh-oh. Do you see what's coming next? How about another study?

"Everyone wanted to measure the fat in our diets," says Lundell. "The primary study on the fat theory was conducted by Ancel Keys of the University of Minnesota. Keyes published the famous and controversial Seven Countries Study in which they concluded that the amount of fat consumed within various worldwide cultures dictated whether those nations were heart-healthy. The study compared populations, such as those in Japan and Crete, who had little heart disease, with those in Finland, which were plagued with it. And, how can you argue with that? All the results made sense with the diets of those populations. People in Finland eat a lot of fatty foods. And, because of that, dietary fat became known as the 'greasy killer.' The next thing you knew is that Keyes was on the cover of *Time* Magazine. Still, nobody was quite sure what effect cholesterol had on the body."

Okay, how many times have we seen this happen in America? We see it all the time. A new finding creates a buzz—all of sudden Jane Fonda is selling oodles of exercise videos, Richard Simmons is revolutionizing the war on obesity, and everyone thinks that a resolution to all their health problems has arrived. Ta-da!

"These studies aren't bad," says Dr. Lundell. "The publicity generated was phenomenal. It brought awareness of heart disease to the forefront—now it was a household discussion. Any health craze in America is a good thing. But, these studies were still missing a big piece of the puzzle. When you miss a big piece, and the epidemic continues to grow, it's time to refocus."

Rest assured, not everyone was on board with the findings from the Framingham or Keyes studies. In fact, many scientists and doctors argued against the findings.

"The studies were controversial," says Lundell. "Numerous scientists argued against the theory of cholesterol and denounced the theory that dietary fat consumption was the cause of heart disease. Nevertheless, the fat/cholesterol diet theory was still gaining popularity in America. So no one paid attention to the facts. Why? Well, that's a great question."

It's controversial. It raises numerous unanswered questions. Science and medicine hadn't even flushed out all the necessary facts to support the fat and cholesterol theory, yet the general public was leaping with great strides to jump on the low-fat bandwagon. Maybe low-fat and low-cholesterol made sense to the American people. Maybe it felt good to limit fat intake. It seemed like it would work. But, heart disease continued to rise—at staggering rates, affecting more people than it ever had in history.

Wow. It'd be great to go home to your significant other at the end of the day, climb into bed, lovingly turn your head with pride and say, "Honey, I followed the new low-fat and low-cholesterol diet plan. I'm making great progress. My heart disease is progressing daily. Soon, I may even get myself one of those heart attacks."

Again, that was sarcasm. But, it's really what was happening in households across the nation. Our country is obsessed with low-fat and low-cholesterol products. And, we're dying.

"They said that a low-fat diet would make you live longer," said Lundell. "Well, it didn't. It only seemed like an eternity. Everything that tasted good was removed from the American diet. That's why everyone went on rollercoaster diets. How long can you survive on a diet that doesn't taste good?"

The low-fat diet tasted horrible. It didn't work. And yet, the United States Government was supporting the theory. It was only a matter of time until they would make it official public policy. Go figure.

"It's interesting," says Dr. Lundell. "In 1968, the United States Senate formed a bipartisan, non-legislative committee on nutrition and human needs, chaired by Senator George McGovern. The committee's goal was to get rid of malnutrition in America. It was a good thing. We need to feed the people, right? But, as the malnutrition focus began to peter out in the mid-70s, the committee didn't disappear. It decided it should address the nutrition of our nation—now it wasn't about feeding the people, it was focused on what we should eat."

Of course, this seemed like a good idea to Senator McGovern and his fellow senators—all middle-aged men who were beginning to worry about their own girth and longevity. Who can blame the Senators? There's a huge health scare amongst a world super power—heart disease is running rampant. Add to that, those groovy hip huggers all the kids were wearing in the 70's didn't compliment a middle-aged spread. By golly, something had to be done.

Call out the scientists!
Let's do something about this disease!

In July of 1976, Senator McGovern's committee listened to two full days of testimony on proposed nutritional standards. The recommendations from that committee suggested that Americans cut their fat intake to less than 30% of calories, and their saturated fat intake to less than 10%. These standards were released in January of 1977. They perfectly reflected the American Heart Association's recommendations for men with a high risk of heart disease.

Again, it seems the recommendations for women were an over-sight—misplaced, or overtly ignored.

"Obviously, the beef, dairy and poultry industries were outraged and lobbied hard against those recommendations," says Lundell. "Beef and dairy products were the leaders in dietary fat. And, we're a nation that likes meat and cheese. Bang! Just like that, people weren't buying these products. This became a lobby war within government—the meat and dairy producers versus the bread and cereal manufacturers. The grain lobbyist loved it."

The battles between the two groups continued. Everyone thought the guidelines might disappear when the committee disbanded in 1977. But, that's not the case.

Maybe the lobbyists were really persistent. Maybe there were a few bucks floating around in the pockets of politicians. Or, maybe the public outcry to find something that worked—just so something was being done—was too much pressure for the government to allow the committee to dissolve.

Roll out the paperwork—the new recommendations would turn into official public policy.

What does it take to create an official public policy? What does it take to make anything official in government? It takes a whole bunch of money.

As early as 1971, a task force for the National Institute of Health estimated that a trial to prove that a low-fat diet actually prolonged life and reduced heart disease would cost $1 billion. Wow, now we're talking politics!

"Politics can get in the way of saving lives," says Lundell. "A real, in-depth study was too much money for the government to consider. They didn't want to spend a billion dollars. So, they opted for smaller studies taking 10 years to finish and costing around $500 million."

This is a mandate that doesn't make sense. Find out how to cure this thing. Do whatever it takes. Just don't spend too much money. A price tag was the presiding factor. It wasn't about finding the truth. It was about maintaining a budget. And, that raised even more questions. Was the money being spent to prove that the low-fat theory was correct? Or were they willing to spend money to discover that it didn't work?

"The studies focused on how cholesterol could be reduced," says Dr. Lundell. "Not whether it actually created a risk of heart disease. In fact, in 1984, the Lipid Research Clinics (LRC) study, a $140 million trial, reported that a medication called cholestyramine reduced cholesterol levels and modestly reduced heart disease in men with abnormally high cholesterol levels. The investigators concluded (without any supporting dietary information) that low-cholesterol dietary recommendations should be extended to the population in general. They felt that they had established the critical link between lowering dietary cholesterol, blood cholesterol and heart disease. This conclusion was made in spite of the fact that it was a drug trial, not a diet trial."

Oh? Here's another bit of sarcasm: A drug trial get used to push diet advice? Why on earth would they do that?

59

Of course, after the LRC results were released, a massive public health campaign was launched. *Time* Magazine's headline read, "Sorry, it's true. Cholesterol really is a killer." The article began by stating, "No whole milk. No butter. No fatty meats." Three months later, *Time* Magazine's cover photo was a frowning face—a breakfast plate with two fried eggs as the eyes, and a down-turned strip of bacon for the mouth.

Wow. That was a sad day for heart disease—frowning egg faces, incomplete science, and a dangerous theory being promoted to millions of unsuspecting Americans.

Later that same year, the National Institute of Health held what they called' a "consensus conference" to justify the LRC study. The concept behind this conference is much like a jury—aligning a supposedly unbiased panel of experts who would listen to testimony and arrive at a conclusion. Just like a jury, every panel member must agree to reach a verdict. During the conference, a few of the 20 experts had demonstrated defects within the studies—they claimed the studies were inaccurate. Nevertheless, the final conference report revealed no disagreement—it was conclusive. Everyone was on the low-fat band-wagon. The final report clearly stated, "There is no doubt that low-fat diets will afford significant protection against coronary heart disease in every American over two years old."

That sealed the deal. The low-fat diet was now official public policy. And, it was about to become one of the most publicized and recognized government policies in history.

Here comes the publicity.

Following that conference, The United States Department of Agriculture issued the famous food pyramid—plastered across the side panel of every box of cereal and crackers that line the isles of our grocery stores. That food pyramid has become reading material at breakfast tables everywhere—and it has dictated the way millions of Americans make daily food choices. Our public school systems even use the pyramid as a guide for nutrition education.

"That's how the low-fat theory turned into dogma," says Dr. Lundell. "Millions of dollars were spent lobbying the various agencies and legislators so that the recommendations became favorable to the industries paying the lobbyists."

Yes, all major food manufacturers have lobbyists fighting for the government's recommendation to promote more consumption of their products on a daily basis. That's one crutch of capitalism— money gets things done.

"How do you like the idea that someone like Jack Abramoff (a political lobbyist and activist who is consistently involved with political scandals) decides what you should eat everyday? It's all about money," says Lundell. "As I mentioned earlier, the beef, dairy, and poultry industries were heavily against the new recommendations. The grain and cereal industries obviously were in favor. The food pyramid suggests 9 to 11 servings of grains and starches every day— that's a lot of support for grain-based foods, and a lot of money. The efforts of lobby groups aren't evil. We just need to keep in mind that lobby groups aren't focusing on anything except gaining governmental support for their industries. That's just how business is done in Washington, DC. But, what does it cost our health?"

When billions of dollars are on the line for food manufacturers, health can take the back seat. Even though the statistics were proving that the low-fat/high carbohydrate diet was actually increasing heart disease in

America, the publicity surrounding the diet continued to woo millions of unsuspecting Americans. And, the more the public buys into a theory, the more our marketing departments advertise that theory.

Low-fat crackers! Low-fat cereal! Low-fat licorice! Let the advertising frenzy begin!

And the advertising messages don't stop in the aisles of our grocery stores. It's human nature to pass along well-publicized information—mothers tell their children, friends tell colleagues, and patterns of belief soon become engrained in culture. Think about it. Some dietary suggestions have even become folklore—more commonly referred to as a wives' tale. Oysters can inspire virility? An apple a day keeps the doctor away? And, a watermelon will grow in your stomach if you swallow a watermelon seed? Some of these dietary tidbits have been floating around for decades without any scientific evidence. If the folklore passes around enough, it becomes public consensus—even if it sounds ridiculous.

"Once a concept becomes public consensus, it's difficult to overcome," says Dr. Lundell. "And, that has been a discussion of philosophers, scientists, and sociologist for a long time. Many are still being discussed today. Yet, they have nothing to do with science. Author Michael Crichton, in a recent book wrote something like this. *Let's be clear: the work of science has nothing whatever to do with consensus. Consensus is the business of politics. Science, on the contrary, requires only one investigator, who happens to be right, which means that he or she has results that are verifiable in the real world.*"

Lundell is right. Crichton is right. Public consensus has no place in science. And, sadly, it seems that science hasn't made its way into public consensus regarding the reality of heart disease.

But, c'mon, are we to blame ourselves? Are we, the public, really influenced by the media? Do we believe the old wife's tales? And, are we too afraid to question public consensus—to challenge it?

"A good example of challenging consensus with fact is the recent Nobel Prize in medicine awarded in 2005," says Lundell. "Australian researchers proposed that a certain type of bacteria was the cause of a stomach ulcer disease. Everything they said challenged public consensus. These researchers were ridiculed, vilified, discredited—called crackpots. But, they had the science. So to prove it, they ultimately performed experiments on themselves by ingesting the bacteria, contracting ulcers, and then curing the ulcers with antibiotics to prove their theory. Since then, they have dramatically altered the treatment of ulcer disease—no more surgery and antacids. Now, the disease is treated with appropriate antibiotics. People think medicine just is what it is—that it shouldn't be challenged. But, all the major breakthroughs have been inspired by someone challenging consensus."

Okay, so Dr. Lundell can challenge consensus. He's a notable heart surgeon. He's a leader in medicine. He's privy to all the right information. Is it possible for the rest of us to change our own perspectives, let alone the consensus of the public?

Do we, the normal people of the world, have enough information to educate our peers? Are we ready to call foul on the low-fat diet? Are we ready to face ridicule by saying cholesterol isn't the culprit?

"The dogma on low-fat diets and cholesterol will continue, in spite of the overwhelming lack of conclusive evidence that they "have any redeeming effect on" to read "have any effect on heart disease reduction," says Lundell. "Low-fat diets have many adverse unintended consequences. But, our country is so engrained in the theory that it will persist. The only way to challenge the dogma is through information. I said it before and I'll continue to repeat myself; anyone who arms themselves with the information in this book can save many hundreds of more lives than I ever could as a heart surgeon."

Wait a second. What about all those studies? When we face the world and call foul on the low-fat diet, won't people backlash with Framingham, LRC, or Keyes? Weren't these good, credible studies?

What makes a good experiment?

Do you still remember your science class? The ideal experiment, as you may recall from whatever lab experience you had in school, is to control all the variables of the experiment except one. It's like growing little trees—the pots are the same, the soil is the same, the sunlight and water are the same, and the air and temperature are the same. To create a valid experiment, you would toss some fertilizer on just one of the plants to see if it makes a difference. Then, you can make observations and conclusions based on the results you achieved by changing that single variable.

A controlled experiment is a good experiment. Sure. All your ducks are in a row. You can monitor a controlled experiment to get the whole story.

Do the same rules apply to an experiment that studies people?

Hmm? How do you control people? As you can imagine, with humans it is impossible to control variables—we all lead different lives, eat different things and have the freedom to make different life choices. It would be almost impossible to control the amount of exercise, sleep, stress, and dietary intake of any human being, much less a group of people. Yes, it's been done in hospital wards where every bit of food and every activity can be completely controlled. But, these can only be short-term experiments. At some point, people will bust out of captivity for a cheeseburger and cigarette, right? Sure they will.

That said, when human beings are studied, it's critically important to design the study so that the answer is not predetermined—people need to live their lives as if they weren't part of a study.

When observing people, the amount of variables that exist in their lives will determine how big the study group needs to be in order to achieve statistical significance. The term Statistical Significance simply means that the results of a study are more likely to reflect the monitored changes that occur during a study, rather than random chance.

Why would you need to understand the definition of *Statistical Significance*? That's simple. Basically that whole paragraph reveals that results of studies aren't random. And, if they're not random, there's a good possibility that the results themselves can be controlled—at least to a certain extent.

Here's an easier description. Have you ever heard a statistic that seemed like it was too good to be true and you said to yourself, "They can fudge those numbers to mean anything they want them to mean?" Well, that's the point—studies can be based on *Statistical Significance*. It's not wrong. It's just not whole.

"In one of the papers I published at Yale about the different methods of preserving the heart muscle during coronary bypass, I proved that one method was superior to another," says Dr. Lundell. "But, to prove the point of how a test can be misleading, we started a trial just after one patient had died and ended the trial just before another patient died. These two deaths could've added two more death records to our mortality rate—that would have changed our overall mortality considerably. But, people never asked about why we started, or why we finished the study when we did. This is common practice in studies, especially when scientists are seeking specific results."

Medicine—fudged to produce more impressive numbers?

Let's revisit the rules of science. The typical way to prove a theory focused on people, is to select two groups who are as similar as possible in characteristics—sex, age, lifestyle, etc. One group is called the control group and carries on as normal, or is given a placebo treatment—a treatment that the control group believes is a treatment, but the treatment really has no effect. The other group is called the intervention group—the 'lab rats' who receive the real drug, or treatment, or lifestyle change.

Then the test is conducted and the two groups are compared to discover the differences—lab rats versus control group.

This is pretty basic stuff—an education most of us learned in science class. Why are we revisiting it at the end of this chapter?

"Throughout this book, I keep referring to the facts," says Lundell. "The most influential and respected investigation into heart disease is the Framingham heart study. And, this is where we need to drill back down to the simple facts. We need to look back to how a proper study is conducted. The Framingham Study was set up by Harvard University Medical School to study a population from Framingham, Massachusetts. More than 5000 people were enrolled in the initial study. Harvard is now studying the second and third generations of these original subjects. This study was not a comparative study. It was simply an observational study. There was no control group and no intervention group. The entire enrollee population was observed. The group's habits, diets, blood pressure activity, and blood cholesterol were all measured and analyzed. But, there's really nothing to compare here—it was simply a gathering of data."

So, that's not a proper experiment?

Lundell continues, "Throughout the study, dietary intake of cholesterol varied over a wide range—everyone consumed different amounts. Yet, no matter how much or how little cholesterol a person in the study consumed, there was little or no difference in cholesterol levels of their blood. Basically, this proves we cannot form a link between the amounts of cholesterol consumed though foods and the amount of cholesterol in the blood. Then, the scientists studied the intakes of saturated fats. Once again, the results showed no relationship to blood cholesterol. It didn't matter how much fat a person ate."

What have we really learned?

"We learned something extremely valuable," says Dr. Lundell. "There's no correlation between the fat we consume and the cholesterol in our blood. And, more than 22 years after the study began, the researchers conducting the study, finally agreed that consumption didn't make a difference by concluding: *"There is, in short, no suggestion of any relation between diet and the subsequent development of chronic heart disease in the study group."*

Plop. There's a whole bunch of results that proved nothing.

Interestingly enough, the research continued—still focusing on cho-lesterol—but concluding with some extremely unexpected results.

"In December of 1997, another follow-up report showed that an increased consumption of saturated fats actually reduced the stroke rate," says Lundell. "That had to be a bad day for those researchers. Not only did they not get what they were expecting, but the results proved opposite."

Wait. If we learned anything from our discussion on biology, we know that a heart attack and a stroke are basically the same thing. And the science is saying that increased levels of dietary fat reduced the incidence of stroke?

"They couldn't just believe their own findings and accept the sci-ence," says Dr. Lundell. "Because strokes typically affect older men, the researchers wondered if a fatty diet was causing people to die of chronic heart disease before they could have a stroke. That statement just goes to show how determined they were to prove that choles-terol was the culprit. Eventually, the researchers discounted this pos-sibility by stating ... *this hypothesis, however, depends on the presence of a strong direct association of fat intake with coronary heart disease. Since we found no direct association, competing mortality from coro-nary heart disease is very unlikely to explain our results.*"

What does all that mumbo jumbo really mean?

"Ha!" laughs Dr. Lundell. "It means that after 49 years of research, there is no association between a fatty diet and heart disease."

The Framingham Study isn't the only study with "disappointing" results when it comes to proving the fat and cholesterol theory.

Here are a few more examples:

MR. FIT Study

The multiple risk factor intervention trial, known as the MR. FIT, cost $115 million, involved 28 medical centers and 250 researchers.

A total of 361,662 men were screened and only those with higher risk for coronary disease were chosen. A total of 12,866 men aged 35 to 57 years were randomly assigned to either an intervention group or usual care group. The intervention group consisted of: increased treatment for hypertension, counseling for cigarette smoking, and dietary advice for lowering blood cholesterol levels. The control group received the usual care in the community. The patients were followed for seven years. The intervention group cut their cholesterol consumption by 42%, saturated fat consumption by 28%. Blood cholesterol levels did fall a modest amount, but overall mortality, and especially mortality from chronic heart disease, was no different in the two groups.

The originators of the study referred to the results as "disappointing".

Their conclusion: "The overall result does not show a beneficial effect on chronic heart disease or total mortality from this multi-factor intervention."

The Physician's Health Study

The Physician's Health Study (PHS) enrolled a total of 51,529 male United States health care professionals. These healthcare professionals filled out periodic questionnaires regarding diet, lifestyle, and any changes in the health status. This study demonstrated a 44% reduction in heart attack by consuming a daily dose of aspirin.

Recently, the report on 43,732 of these professionals demonstrated that intake of total fat, cholesterol or specific types of fat had no association or correlation with stroke.

Their conclusion: Dietary fat and cholesterol showed no association with stroke. However, adding a daily dose of aspirin significantly reduced risk regardless of diet.

The Women's Health Initiative Study

The Women's Health Initiative (WHI), which has now cost over $415 million, studied 48,835 postmenopausal women. The groups were randomly assigned to receive no intervention (as the control group) or receive intervention. The intervention group received intensive behavior modification and instruction with the goal of reducing fat intake to 20% calories, increasing consumption of vegatables and fruits to five servings a day, and grains to at least six servings a day. After a mean follow-up of 8.1 years, there was no reduction in the risk of heart disease, stroke, or cancer.

Their conclusion: Following a diet that closely resembles the standard food pyramid showed no reduction of heart disease, stroke, or cancer.

So, let's summarize.

- Reducing intake of cholesterol has no effect on the risk of chronic heart disease.

- Low-fat diets do not reduce the risk of chronic heart disease.

- A daily dose of aspirin (anti-inflammatory) does reduce the risk of chronic heart disease.

How did we end up smack dab in the middle of an epidemic? It seems public consensus and narrowly focused experiments have led us astray from the one thing that could save our lives—the facts.

"All research teaches us something," says Dr. Lundell. "The amazing thing about the studies we discussed here is that they didn't see the real value of their results. It wasn't that these studies didn't prove anything. These studies simply proved that what they were expecting to happen didn't happen. And, that something else must be the cause of heart disease."

What can we do with all this information? Well, to start, we can use the one piece of information included in this chapter that doesn't tell the story of how we ended up in the middle of an epidemic—rather, it provides science to tell us how to climb out.

"Ironically, a huge breakthrough appeared in one of the studies that was overlooked," says Dr. Lundell. "Aspirin has been around a lot longer than any of these studies. But we've had our eyes so narrowly focused on stuff that doesn't matter that the function of a simple aspirin—the reduction of inflammation—was ignored. It's about time we move away from consensus. We need to look at the facts. We need to ask questions. And, when we have the guts to challenge the consensus, we'll see overwhelming results.")(

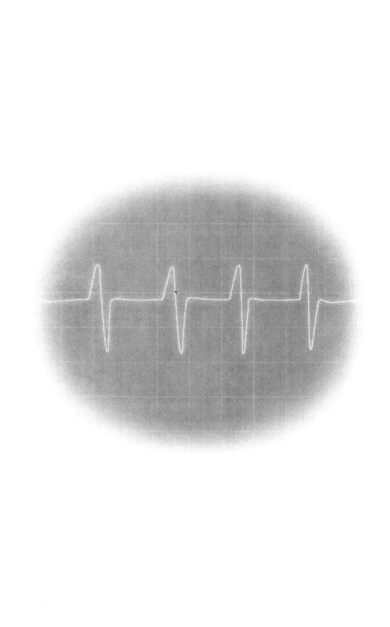

Cause and Defect

What has the low-fat diet done to America?

EVERY ACTION HAS A REACTION. That makes sense. Now, here's what doesn't make sense.

Some of you reading this may still be questioning whether the low-fat and low-cholesterol diets are truly causing an epidemic in America. How can all these sources that promote low-fat diets be wrong?

"There's nothing wrong with low-fat," says Dr. Lundell. "The problems lie in the recommendations to exclusively avoid fat. Just because a food is low-fat, doesn't make it healthy—for the heart or the entire body."

The diet-heart theory has been around for nearly a century. It began when rabbits were fed a diet high in cholesterol and saturated fats. As a result of this diet, they developed fatty deposits in their blood vessels. Researchers at the time thought they had found a direct correlation between high fat diets and arteriosclerosis. And, why wouldn't they look further into the theory—it seemed like a rational explanation.

"I'm not promoting fat," says Dr. Lundell. "I'm simply proposing that the current epidemic is caused by other culprits. Fatty foods don't make people fat. High cholesterol diets don't cause heart disease. The recommendations need to change."

But, doesn't it seem like recommendations are always changing anyway? You can't turn on a television news magazine anymore without seeing a story about obesity in America. And, although this book is not focused on obesity, the issue needs to be discussed.

"Excessive body fat is an indicator of heart disease," says Dr. Lundell. "This isn't just a statistic that says that overweight people have a higher tendency to have heart disease. We have the science that shows the biology—body fat increases inflammation."

Oh, so obesity is not like cholesterol? It's not just a number tallied as some sort of common denominator—here's the number of obese people and here's the number of people with chronic heart disease? There's actually a biological link?

"Today, we can show how fatty tissues cause chronic low-grade inflammation," says Dr. Lundell. "And, sadly, a large percentage of Americans believe that if they cut the fat in their diet, they'll cut the fat around their waist line. It's simply not true."

Just to prove Dr. Lundell's last statement, consider the shelves of your grocery store. You can buy regular potato chips, light potato chips, reduced fat potato chips, fat blocking potato chips, and fat free potato chips. The same goes for other products on the shelves. And, every year a new product comes to market that claims to even have lower fat than all its competitors.

The fat content in foods continues to decrease. Yet, our belt lines continue to increase. And, the entire time you think you're doing something good for yourself, you're really just suffering through a bag of cardboard-tasting potato chips.

Almost all manufactured food products have a low-fat version nowadays. And, many of these 'fat-tailored' options have been around for decades. So, why does our nation continue to gain weight?

"It's a confusing mess," says Dr. Lundell. "In spite of the fact that there was no evidence to support the low-fat theory, it continues to be the focus. Everyone is screaming for change. And, instead of looking at the low-fat theory and its results on the American public, food manufacturers just continue lowering the fat content. The lower it gets, the fatter we become."

Hmm? The fat content in foods gets lower, while the nation gets fatter? What about the good old slogan, "You are what you eat?" Is that wrong?

"It is wrong," says Lundell. "Instead of focusing on what we put inside our bodies, we need to focus on what our bodies do with the foods we consume—what happens when those foods enter the metabolic process. The U.S. Department of Agriculture (USDA) adopted the now famous food pyramid and began a public health campaign to change the diet of America. Well, guess what? It's not working. It's not making our nation thinner and healthier and it's not reducing the incidence of heart disease. As we have also discussed, elevated blood cholesterol levels are associated with heart disease. But, remember, association does not equal cause."

He's right. What if all banjo players in America were studied and a large percentage of those people had developed heart disease? Would we recommend reduced banjo plucking? Fatty foods don't necessarily equal fatty bodies. And, cholesterol doesn't equal heart disease. They simply share a common denominator—which has nothing to do with biology.

"We need facts in this battle, not faith," says Dr. Lundell. "When it was demonstrated that cholesterol-lowering drugs lowered blood cholesterol, researchers made an unfortunate leap of faith. They assumed that if lowering cholesterol by medication was effective against heart disease, reducing fat intake would also lower cholesterol and reduce coronary disease. I have no criticism of faith for a religion. But, why are we taking a leap of faith when it comes to science? It doesn't make sense. This is something we can cure. You can stop heart disease in its tracks."

So, there's a lot of wishful finger-crossing going on in America—hoping for a possible benefit from the low-fat and low-cholesterol theory. The National Institutes of Health, the National Cholesterol Education Program, the American Heart Association, the US Department of Agriculture, and a host of other medical organizations are joining the food industry to promote and publicize the low-fat diet—hoping we'll get lucky and the statistics will suddenly change direction.

Is this a conspiracy theory? Are they trying to trick us?

"It's not a conspiracy," says Dr. Lundell. "It's simply a tired theory— a notion that has turned into consensus. The problem is that this consensus is based on incomplete science. All these groups have good intentions. But, look at the facts. When will the public, the politicians, the medical organizations, and the food manufacturers start waving their white flags and surrender to science? I admitted that I was wrong, why can't they?"

Our supermarket shelves are filled with every imaginable low-fat product, including cookies, cakes, ice cream, milk and bread—all of them are marked prominently on their labels as "low-fat." And, as consumers, it's almost impossible to ignore the 'low-fat' labels and get at least a little excited about the fact that a bag of cookies has half the fat as its counterpart. C'mon, that means we can eat double the cookies, right?

What message does 'low-fat' send to the consumer?

"The message the manufacturers are sending is unmistakable," says Dr. Lundell. "Eat all the low-fat food you want. It's safe. We can eat all we want and still be healthy. That's simply false. And, it's dangerous."

Yeah; Oops. We're not healthy.

Today, brand name foods exist on the shelves that were created simply to fill the niche of the low-fat craze. And, it's easy to see why these brands arose—there was a huge demand. Huge demands equal enormous profit. It seems brilliant—create a food that tastes like a snack, yet make it seemingly healthy. Cha-ching—the sound of cash registers clanking all across America.

"A low-fat brand generates enormous profits," says Dr. Lundell. "Snackwell® cookies come to mind. This is great business. It's too bad that branding broccoli as a low-fat food doesn't create the same profits. Why aren't all vegetables labeled so prominently with the low-fat label?"

Hey, why aren't they branded as health foods? Most canned vegetables just have a simple picture and the ingredients—where's all the marketing sizzle? Why don't we see words like "Heart Healthy Snack" on the side of an artichoke? Or, wouldn't it be nice to see our children run to the produce section because their favorite super hero or princess is stuck to it?

If cutting the fat out of our diets is truly the answer, wouldn't vegetables be a good start? There's an advertising campaign we can stand behind to cut the fat. But, obviously that's not the focus.

The focus of the current recommendations is to cut the fat in foods that, for one reason or another, started off as unhealthy. We only see low-fat labels on the stuff we shouldn't eat anyway. And, food manufacturers have responded with overwhelming vigor.

The question is: are we consuming less fat because of the advertising?

The answer is: yes. Over the past 25 years, the percent of calories consumed as fat has dropped significantly. The average serum cholesterol has dropped as well. There's no doubt that the campaign worked and is still working. Americans consume less fat. Perfect. Or, not perfect?

"Of course the campaign worked," says Lundell. "Look at the results. If proponents want to stand up and say that their low-fat campaign worked, they'll all look like superstars. Of course, that's if their goal was to reduce the consumption of fat—which it was. However, if their goal was to reduce obesity or heart disease, it's a completely different story. Then the campaign would be a royal flop."

Obesity rates in the United States remained stable at around 14 or 15% from 1900 to 1980. Since then, the obesity rates have skyrocketed. Today, nearly 60% of the population is overweight or obese. If you toss those numbers onto a chart, you'll see the huge spike in the number of obese people in America—it's so dramatic that you'd think our nation declared a free-for-all eating festival.

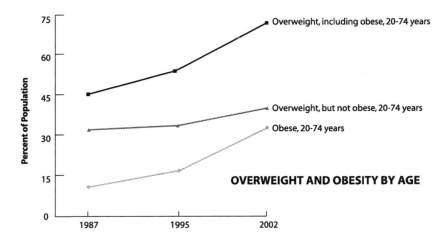

The irony, of course, is that the spike in the number of obese Americans began and progressed as the government recommended the opposite of a free-for-all feast—the spike happened when they reduced the recommended fat in our diet.

Now we have a double-edged sword—food packaging says eat less fat, and the media continues to air stories about how fat we've become. At first the obesity epidemic was somewhat of a side show attraction—a curiosity of a population outgrowing airline seats and standard clothing sizes. But now, it's become much more serious. Being overweight or obese doesn't just affect your pants size anymore.

Today, obesity has a direct link to type II diabetes (adult onset diabetes). People with type II diabetes do not produce enough insulin for the amount of sugar they consume. It's that, or their cells simply ignore the insulin (often referred to as *insulin* resistant). Insulin is necessary for the body to be able to use sugar. Type II diabetes rates have continued to spike dramatically over the past decade, and the disease is now showing up as early as adolescence. In fact, each year it seems the onset of the disease continues to strike at an earlier age.

If that's not bad enough, a new disease has appeared on the scene, which has been linked to diet and obesity. It's called Syndrome X or Metabolic Syndrome, which is now present in 40% of middle-aged American adults. Metabolic Syndrome is characterized by an increase in abdominal fat, blood fat disorders, insulin resistance, and elevated blood pressure.

Type II diabetes, and Metabolic Syndrome have been headlining stories lately on television and in our newspapers. You've seen and read the stories. You've seen John Stossel asking the questions that most of us fear. And, you've seen the obligatory camera shots of overweight people strolling down the sidewalk somewhere in America. Stossel is asking the questions. He is challenging the current recommendations. Still, the epidemic continues to flourish. And, the television ratings must flourish for these fat-focused programs as well—we see a new one every couple of months.

Is there an end to the fat? And, what exactly does this have to do with heart disease?

"Remember, we're made up of living cells," says Dr. Lundell. "Everything in your body is connected. Diabetes and Metabolic Syndrome are major risk factors for coronary artery disease. These diseases are caused by obesity. And, these diseases are directly linked to diet."

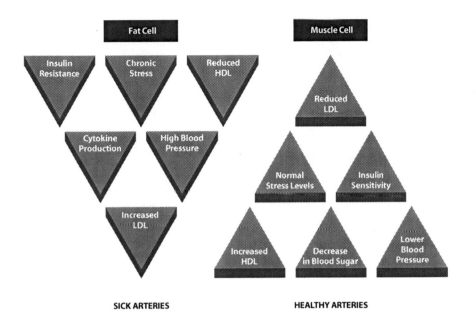

The list doesn't stop there. Many diseases are directly linked to diet. In fact, most diseases are linked to diet. If you recall the discussion we had earlier about inflammation and how your body's own defense system rallies when a certain part of the body is fighting an infection, consider all the inflammatory responses that could be happening if you're battling your weight, if you're battling excessive pressure on your joints, and if you're lacking in necessary nutrients.

According to the American Obesity Association, adults and children who suffer from obesity are at high risk of developing the following medical conditions. As you read through the list of conditions that can be tied directly to obesity, just keep in mind that every cell is connected in your body.

Obesity-Related Medical Conditions Include:
- Arthritis
- Osteoarthritis (OA)
- Rheumatoid Arthritis (RA)
- Birth Defects
- Cancers:
  o Breast Cancer
  o Cancers of the Esophagus and Gastric Cardia
  o Colorectal Cancer
- Cardiovascular Disease (CVD)
- Carpal Tunnel Syndrome (CTS)
- Chronic Venous Insufficiency (CVI)
- Daytime Sleepiness
- Deep Vein Thrombosis (DVT)
- Diabetes (Type II)
- End Stage Renal Disease (ESRD)
- Gallbladder Disease
- Gout
- Heat Disorders
- Hypertension
- Impaired Immune Response
- Impaired Respiratory Function
- Infections Following Wounds
- Liver Disease
- Low Back Pain
- Obstetric and Gynecologic Complications
- Chronic Pain
- Pancreatitis
- Sleep Apnea
- Stroke
- Surgical Complications
- Urinary Stress Incontinence

Most of you didn't read that entire list. And, that's okay. The list is provided simply to illustrate how one health condition can lead to a host of other conditions. Nevertheless, if there is one thing you should know about the long list of ailments, it's this: Inflammation is the common factor in almost every single one!

It's kind of like that one toxic employee at your workplace. Just one bad attitude can create numerous problems, complaints, and headaches. One bad employee can create a contagious negative energy throughout the entire organization. Pretty soon, work production is down, company morale is down, and profits are down. If it's bad enough, the entire business could end up closing its doors. Kaput. Done.

Easy fix? It may appear that way at first. If this discussion focused on a toxic personality, it would be easy to scream, "They deserve to be fired!" If that person were fired, would all the problems disappear? Would your workplace be happy? It could be. But, what if management kept recommending bad employees to fill that new empty position? Then what?

Compare this situation to the human body. If the recommendations are wrong, then what do we do?

"I've been saying all along that we're not talking about one part of the body," says Dr. Lundell. "Yes, we're battling heart disease, but it doesn't do us any good to just look at the heart. We've got to go back to the root of the problem. We've got to start from scratch. We've got to see where the issue truly begins in the biological process."

If we were actually talking about a toxic coworker, the trail of toxicity would need to be traced all the way back to that person's initial employment. Did a hiring manager simply hire the wrong person? Did they not check references?

Heart disease—let's backtrack.

What has changed?

"There's only one thing that has changed," says Dr. Lundell. "It's not us. Analysis of DNA evidence reveals that there has been very little change in the human genome over the past 10,000 years. We're the same biological creatures. The only change has been lifestyle and dietary habits. And, the greatest change—the largest increase in obesity and heart disease has occurred in the past few decades with the low-fat diet."

Is he saying that our genetics are still the same? Doesn't our heredity have anything to do with this epidemic? Aren't we morphing into some sort of genetically dysfunctional species?

"Nope," says Lundell. "Genetically, we're the same. A modern example of similar genealogy is the Pima Indian living in Arizona compared to the Pima Indian living in Mexico. The Arizona Pima has the highest rate of diabetes, kidney failure and obesity in the country. The Pima Nation has been studied extensively because the numbers are so extreme. The Pima Indians in Arizona have adopted a Western lifestyle and diet—they have fast food chains and grocery store shelves lined with low-fat cookies just like the rest of us."

Here's the catch.

"The other portion of the Pima Indian Nation remained in Mexico, living a rural lifestyle. Diabetes, kidney failure, obesity and heart disease are almost unknown in this group of genetically identical people—they're from the same small group of ancestry."

Same people. Toxic food choices.

What has caused a toxic environment in America?

"We dedicated the entire last chapter focusing on how the current low-fat recommendations came into effect," says Dr. Lundell. "We discussed the lobby groups and the financial gain of the food industries. We discussed the studies and how they didn't examine every facet because they were too narrowly focused or didn't have enough funding. We've discussed the fact that the low-fat diet doesn't equal a low-fat population. And, we've discussed how all cells are connected—one cell impacts another in any biological process."

Okay, Dr. Lundell, so what's the point?

"If the low-fat and low-cholesterol diet isn't causing obesity and heart disease, what is?" he asks. "It's time to look at the real science. Let's find out where this epidemic really began. Let's find out what is really killing us. Let's find out how we can get control."

Well, here's the part you already know. Today most of us dwell in a mechanized urban setting, leading largely sedentary lives. Let's face it, for a lot of us, a brisk walk only happens when we head to the washroom after our second cup of coffee.

If we're not eating so much fat anymore, what are we eating?

That's easy. We're eating a highly processed synthetic low-fat/high carbohydrate diet. We eat starches—breads, pastas, potatoes, rice, crackers, and cereals. And, we also consume oodles of sugar, which by the way, is often packaged as "fat free".

What's happening to our biology when we eat these foods in mass quantities?

"The simple answer is what we've been talking about in this chapter," says Lundell. "We're getting fat from low-fat."

Two thirds of Americans are overweight or obese. The lifetime incidence of hypertension is an astounding 90%. Cardiovascular disease remains the number one cause of death in the United States and is expected to double in the next 50 years, because of the projected increased rate of obesity and diabetes.

Some authors have called this trend of health deterioration an "affluenza"—meaning it's a result of our affluence. Basically, we can afford to get fat and sick. Others have called it a disease of convenience—we eat whatever tastes good and is easiest to grab. But, here's another thought: we could also call this a disease of lethargy—meaning the vicious circle of unhealthy habits makes us less and less able to do anything about it. Are we couch potatoes because we're lazy? Or, has our diet provided us with less energy to get up and exercise?

Does anyone remember the hunter and gatherer?

"Let's look back a little more than 10,000 years at our ancestors," says Dr. Lundell. "Remember, our ancestors share a virtually identical genome."

Historical and archaeological evidence shows that hunters and gatherers were generally lean, fit, and largely free from signs and symptoms of chronic diseases. That makes perfect sense. They could track an animal for days before they ever got close enough to catch it and call it dinner. That's a lot of exercise. But, why were they virtually free of chronic disease? Was it the hunting or gathering? Or, was it the meal afterward?

"It's a combination of all three," says Dr. Lundell. "But, let's really dig deep. Realize that long before technological advances, all of our ancestors exercised a great deal in their average life—they didn't have cars, or matches to light fires, or water flowing out of taps. They still worked very hard to accomplish simple tasks that we take for granted. Yet, history shows that when hunters and gatherers transitioned to an agricultural grain based diet, their health generally deteriorated."

Archeological studies of bones and teeth have revealed that populations who changed to a grain-based diet didn't grow as tall, had a shorter life span, higher childhood mortality, and a higher incidence of osteoporosis and rickets—along with numerous other mineral and vitamin deficiency diseases.

In recent history, the Pima Indian Nation is a good example, when hunting and gathering societies adopted western lifestyles, kidney failure, atherosclerosis, and obesity become commonplace—in some circumstances record-breaking.

"Obviously, we have not adapted well to a low-fat high carbohydrate diet," says Dr. Lundell. "Can we adapt? It's possible, but it may take another 10,000 years. I don't have that long to wait. And, at the current increasing rate of heart disease and other chronic diseases, I don't think our country will make it that long. We need to change our thinking. We need to change it now."

Is the publicity over the low-fat diet too powerful to overcome? Are the lobbyists and food manufacturers too persuasive? Will the U.S. Government support—and adequately fund—in-depth studies to finally change public consensus?

Or, is it us against them—those of us who know the facts, battling against those who act on faith alone?

"Someday, someone will break the silence and create a huge impact," says Lundell. "My hope is that it starts not with a political figure, or a food manufacturer, or even a doctor like myself. My hope is that a revolution begins with each and every one of us—taking control of an epidemic one life at a time. Start with your own health. Prove it. And, then share the possibilities. Share the power. I said it before—the great thing about biology is that you can change it. Here, we're talking about the biology of an epidemic. That kind of change needs to happen one life at a time. It starts with you."

Once again, Lundell makes a great point. One person may not be able to change the overwhelming consensus of a public misinformed. However, if each of us change our own perspective, and learn from those who have revealed the facts, an epidemic could be ousted.

"The battle isn't new," says Lundell. "There's evidence from the past few years and evidence from more than 100 years ago that the low-fat diet should be challenged. In 2004, Sylvain Lee Weinberg MD, wrote in the Journal of American College of Cardiology, *The low-fat diet heart hypothesis has been the subject of controversy for nearly 100 years. The low-fat high-carbohydrate diet, promulgated vigorously by the National Cholesterol Education Program, National Institutes of Health, and American Heart Association, since the Lipid Research Clinics (LRC) primary prevention program in 1984, and ear-*

lier by the US Department of Agriculture food pyramid, may well have played an unintended role in the current epidemics of obesity, lipid abnormalities, and Metabolic Syndromes. This diet can no longer be defended by appeal to the authority of prestigious medical organizations or by rejecting clinical experience and a growing medical literature suggesting that the much maligned low-carbohydrate-high protein may have a salutary effect on the epidemics in question.

What does that mean?

"That means we're in this predicament for a reason," says Lundell. "That means that we can clearly see where we went wrong. And, that means that there's a simple solution to this problem. The solution has been right in front of us for more than a century. If you want to really know how far back the evidence has existed, you can look at William Banting's Letter on Corpulence, drafted in May of 1869. In that letter, Banting details his own diet, and tracks the overwhelming results. Here's a guy who lowered his cholesterol by eating eggs for breakfast every day. The theory is right there. It just seems to continually be overlooked. But, we can't overlook this anymore. How can we not see it? The further we chase the low-fat diet, the further our nation falls into turmoil?"

Turmoil may be an understatement—especially considering just how easy the solution is to prevent heart disease.

If you have an instant craving for some low-fat potato chips, cookies, crackers, or snacks right about now, you may want to continue reading first.

You just saw what happens when our nation eats a low-fat diet. Now ask yourself; how do we stop it? What are we doing to fix our hearts?

"This is where we stop the inflammation," says Lundell. "This is where we stop the epidemic—starting with you.")(

Surgery, Stents and Statins: Bandages for Heart Disease

WILL SOMEBODY PLEASE DO SOMETHING about the heart disease epidemic in America?

Without question, the United States has the most advanced medical system in the world. Through advances in medical technology and pharmacology, our nation's doctors and health care providers have been able to dramatically reduce the death rates from heart disease—fewer people who have a heart attack will actually die from it.

That sounds like good news. Is it?

"Of course it's good news," says Dr. Lundell. "The sad part of that equation is that we're simply viewing a percentage. Sure, we've been able to reduce the death rate, but we haven't been able to make any progress in reducing the number of people who get coronary disease. In fact, that number continues to rise—at a terrifying rate."

Yes, the numbers continue to get worse every year. And, although different sources may report slightly different numbers, all have one common denominator—the number of people who get heart disease in America is rising drastically and is expected to more than double in the next 50 years.

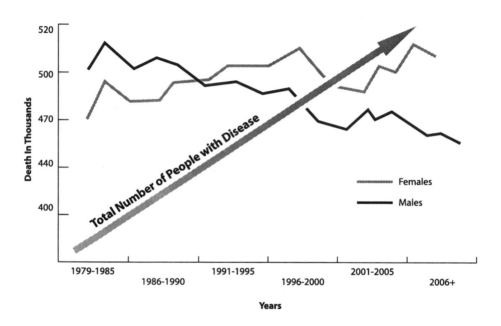

The American Heart Association publishes annual statistics of heart disease and stroke. In the 2006 report, 71,300,000 people in the United States have cardiovascular disease and 13,200,000 have coronary artery disease. There are 700,000 new heart attacks reported annually. And, 5.5 million people have had a stroke, with 700,000 new strokes reported annually. Those numbers may be difficult to comprehend and internalize. But, if we consider the current overall population of approximately 300 million people, those humongous numbers might make a bit more sense—almost 25% are reported to have heart disease.

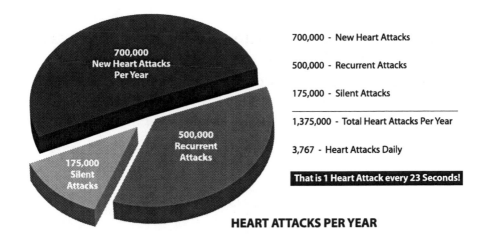

700,000 - New Heart Attacks

500,000 - Recurrent Attacks

175,000 - Silent Attacks

1,375,000 - Total Heart Attacks Per Year

3,767 - Heart Attacks Daily

That is 1 Heart Attack every 23 Seconds!

HEART ATTACKS PER YEAR

"I recently read that the three major industries in the United States are health care, fast food, and then the diet and exercise industry—most likely the fad diets," says Dr. Lundell. "Those are the big money makers. So, what does that tell us?"

Obviously, that tells us that we're a nation who, at least subconsciously, is looking for a solution to our bad habits. We eat. We diet. We eat again. We diet again. And, when the diets don't keep us out of the drive-through window, we seek medical attention to find resolution to our bad choices.

"We're on this bad rollercoaster ride of fad diet trends and junk food which ends up leading to heart disease—the leading killer of Americans since 1990," says Dr. Lundell. "In fact, if you look at the list of the top five causes of death, heart disease almost causes more deaths than the next four causes combined."

Heart disease is the leading killer of women, far exceeding breast-cancer. Among all people between the ages 35 to 44, 20% have been diagnosed with heart disease. 36% of Americans between the ages 45 to 54 have been diagnosed with heart disease. And, among people between 55 to 64 years of age, 55% have been diagnosed with heart disease. By the time the average American reaches the age range of 65 to 74, a whopping 70% will have heart disease. Add to this the number of people who have heart disease and don't know about it yet, and you can see that almost all of us will have problems. It's terrifying."

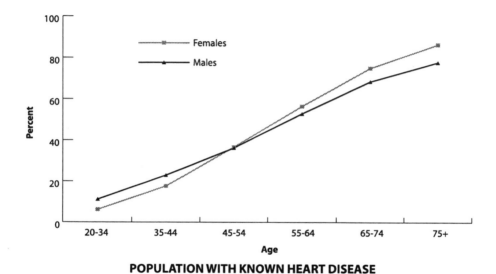

POPULATION WITH KNOWN HEART DISEASE

So, what are we doing about it? Apparently, we're looking for a superhero to save us. As a nation, we're doing nothing about it except crossing our fingers—waiting for the medical community to flex its super muscles and find a magic solution to the problem.

Oh and here's something else to consider: If the current medical establishment is our version of Superman—swooping in at the last second to save our lives—our super hero would send us a bill for $403 billion dollars. That's the price tag for treating heart disease in 2006 alone.

"Modern medicine is good at saving lives," says Dr. Lundell. "The problem is that the number of doctors isn't growing proportionately with the rate of heart disease. Nevertheless, medical technology does continue to improve. Today, the medical community basically uses three therapies to treat the disease—surgery, stents and statins."

Surgery

"The idea of bypassing the blockage in a coronary artery goes back to at least 1910," says Dr. Lundell. "In the 30s and 40s, indirect bypass was attempted by bringing other tissues close to the heart and hoping that small vessels would develop. In 1946, a Canadian surgeon by the name of Vineberg inserted the internal mammary artery from the chest wall into a tunnel in the heart muscle. And, to some degree, his procedure actually enjoyed moderate success in reducing symptoms of inadequate blood flow to the heart muscle. Other surgeons continued to work on methods of directly supplying new blood flow into the coronary artery beyond any obstruction. The most notable of these were Dr. DeBakey of Texas, Dr. Rene Favalaro of the Cleveland Clinic, and Dr. Dudley Johnson of Milwaukee. Of course, if you compare their methods to today's standards, the procedures were crude. But, the work of any pioneer seems crude at first glance, until you can calculate the progress that was made. And, progress is slow at first, but daring and persistent surgeons continued working hard to improve the procedure. With the knowledge they had at the time, these seemingly crude surgeries were the only way to relieve the symptoms of narrowed coronary arteries. Gradually, with the addition and improvement of the heart-lung machine, complications were reduced. By the mid-70s, when I was in surgical training, surgery appeared to be the only effective treatment of coronary artery disease."

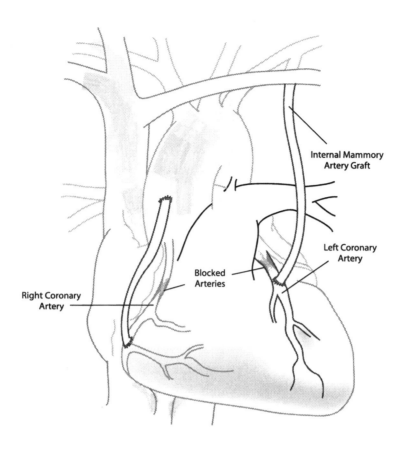

Even today, coronary bypass operation remains a very important treatment method for people with advanced coronary artery disease.

"Sometimes, surgery is still necessary," says Dr. Lundell. "There are certain conditions in which a coronary bypass operation will undoubtedly prolong life. There are also circumstances where a coronary bypass operation will dramatically change a patient's quality of life. I found this aspect—improving the quality of life—especially rewarding during my surgical career. When a person would come in to the hospital with chest pain so severe that they had difficulty going to the bathroom, and we could perform a coronary bypass operation so they could return to work, or resume a hobby, or simply begin to enjoy their life again, it was extremely rewarding. It was the driving force in my career."

The purpose of this book is to prevent you from being in the horrible circumstance of facing a major life-threatening operation. Even though open-heart surgery is practiced today with extreme success, it is still dangerous. The recovery time is long. It's painful. And, it's really pricey!

In 2006, the American Heart Association report estimated 467,000 coronary bypass operations were performed with an average cost of $83,919 per surgery.

"Can we avoid surgery?" asks Dr. Lundell. "That's the new focus driving my career today. I want to help eliminate the risks. I want to eliminate the painful recoveries. And, I want to eliminate the cost. I want to help eliminate the disease altogether!"

Stents

The American Heart Association reports that 1,414,000 cardiac catheterizations were performed in 2003. 664,000 patients had angioplasty. 84% of these had stents inserted.

You've heard those words before—cardiac catheterization, angioplasty, and stent. These fancy words have become typical conversation pieces of the health segment of your nightly news. But, for most people, even though they recognize these words because of their recent publicity, the words don't mean anything.

"There has been a ton of publicity in this area," says Dr. Lundell. "We're all concerned about heart disease and we're all fascinated with high technology solutions. We like the magical quick fixes to problems. The rapid advances in technology, and the publicity to support and promote those advances, have been driven by the device industry (the makers of catheters, balloons, and stents) because they recognized the appeal of a less invasive procedure. Anything less invasive on the human body would lead to rapid growth in the market for their products. Companies also understand that if a tool is easier to use and achieves better results, they could become the market leader—which leads to financial superiority as well. Because of this fact, the history of change in cardiology (the study of the heart and its function) is more dramatic than the change in cardiac surgery."

"Advancements that are driven by business and money, are still advancements," says Dr. Lundell. "Advancement is always good. And, medicine has come a long way in the last fifty years. In the 1950s, 60s, and even into the 70s, the only tools a cardiologist had was an ancient drug called digitalis, some simple diuretics to help get rid of excess fluid, and nitroglycerin to try to reduce chest pain. Cardiologists were diagnostic experts. They had entire textbooks written about analyzing the heart sounds with a simple stethoscope. And, if a patient had chest pains, the presumed cause was narrowed coronary arteries. That presumption was based on the fact that people who died with chest pains actually had narrowed coronary arteries. In some circumstances, an EKG would help to show that the heart muscle was starving for blood. Ultrasound, at the time, was in its infancy. Nuclear medicine was just an idea—without much support. And, cardiac catheterization was a dangerous and complex procedure involving stopping the heart and manually changing x-ray plates. Basically, there weren't too many options to feel good about."

"But, every bit of practice leads to new advances," Dr. Lundell continued. "In the mid-1960s at the Cleveland Clinic, Dr. Mason Sones developed a technique of injecting dye or contrast material directly into the coronary artery. This dramatic advance, using a long flexible catheter, allowed cardiologist to have a direct view of the coronary artery system. Can you imagine the impact? All of a sudden, they could identify the exact place and severity of the narrowing. Now, the decision as to which therapy to provide was much easier. More accurate diagnosis led to the explosive growth of treatment of coronary artery disease by coronary bypass surgery. The progress was significant. Now a cardiologist was not only armed with a stethoscope and skills of observation, but they could get a direct view of the arteries."

Oh, but there was still one minor issue: even if a cardiologist could pinpoint a problem, what could they do about it?

"This is where the frenzy begins—where we start to see real results," says Dr. Lundell. "Up until this point, a cardiologist had no real therapeutic tools except medication. This changed in 1974, when Dr. Andreas Gruentzig, practicing in Europe, inserted a small sausage shaped balloon into the opening of a narrowed artery and then inflated the balloon to reduce the narrowing. That was the first human angioplasty."

Angioplasty is one of those words that everyone knows, but no one knows how to define it. Basically, the word *angio* means artery, and the word *plasty* means change.

"In 1978, the first coronary angioplasty was performed in the United States," says Dr. Lundell. "And it seemed like a great option to surgery. Coronary balloon angioplasty that stretched the opening in a plaque could be done while a patient was awake. Patients could actually go home the next day. Obviously, this was a more appealing treatment than a huge incision and a seven-day hospital stay. But, that didn't mean angioplasty was always safe. Balloon angioplasty, at the time, required emergency surgery in about 10% of the patients. And, about 50% of the time, the narrowing would come back in less than a year. That 're-narrowing' process was called re-stenosis, and it was the Achilles' heel of angioplasty."

Obviously, if the artery is returning to its narrowed state, there's a problem. No one wants to go back into the hospital once a year to have their artery stretched. But, that still wasn't the main issue. Remember our discussion on inflammation?

"Cardiologists began to attack this problem," says Dr. Lundell. "Considerable time and money was invested to study the cellular mechanisms of restenosis. Some experts thought it was just elastic recoil, but under the microscope, it was discovered that the balloon stretching the artery actually caused an injury. So just like we already learned, the healing process or scar formation was the reason the arteries were closing again."

Sheesh! There it was—the culprit was right in front of them. No one was considering a biological solution to inflammation!

"Well, guess what happened next?" asks Lundell. "A mechanical solution was invented to solve a biological problem. The mechanical solution was a small tube of expanded metal mesh, which was inserted into the artery when it was in a collapsed position. Then, by using an angioplasty balloon, it was opened. This metal mesh held the artery open better than a plain angioplasty, but the healing process still brought a high incidence of restenosis."

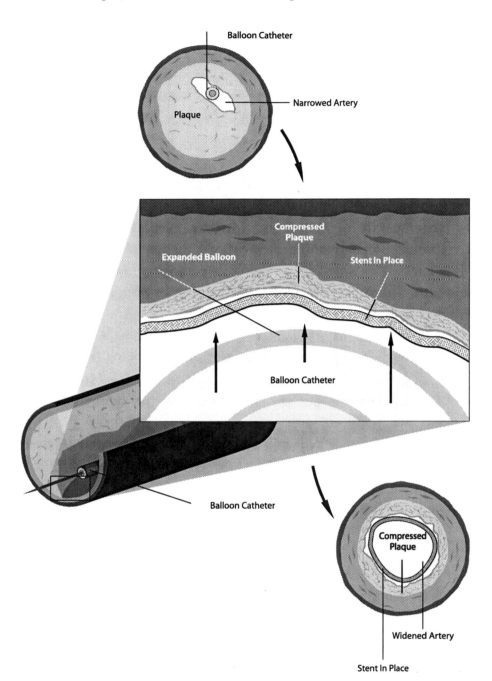

So, the experts went back to the drawing board. This time, the solution was chemical—they bonded a chemical to the metal, which would reduce restenosis. The chemical prevented the healing process from occurring—it hindered the natural healing process. And, the device was approved by the FDA in 2003. It is called a drug eluting stent."

"Of course, stopping the natural healing process comes with a price of its own," adds Dr. Lundell. "Drug-eluting stents had indeed reduced the rate of restenosis. However, every patient with the stent needs blood-thinning medications for the rest of their life. Yes, I guess it's a small price to pay when your other option might be death. But still, reports of sudden death in patients with drug eluting stents have been alarming. When the blood thinning medication is stopped for other elective surgery, new problems arise. At Yale University, for example, patients are brought into the hospital a week ahead of their surgery—no longer is the process an overnight stay. While they are at the hospital, the medications are stopped and replaced with intravenous blood thinners until the time of surgery. Other centers have simply left the patient on their blood thinning medications and accepted the fact that additional blood transfusions would be needed."

So far, none of this sounds very appealing if you're considering quality of life. And, even though this type of aggressive treatment might be necessary, it sure makes you stop and think about the possibility of avoiding it in the first place.

"Stents are certainly overused at this point in time," says Dr. Lundell. "It's frustrating to me to think about it, especially when we can prevent this all from happening. The perception is completely backward. In fact, some cardiologists have developed the mentality of "see narrowing - stent narrowing." They have become enamored by stenting every narrowing—even if it's minimal. This mentality ignores several facts. First, not every narrowing restricts blood flow enough to be a problem. Second, some plaques are stable and are converted to an unstable situation by the insertion of a stent. And third, except in limited circumstances, there is no evidence that stenting prolongs the life. Lost in the middle of all of this hoopla is any significant discussion about preventing coronary artery disease."

Still, Dr. Lundell says that angioplasty and stenting are magnificent procedures in the event of a heart attack.

"If a patient arrives at the emergency room soon after the onset of heart attack symptoms, and they receive the proper diagnosis of a heart attack, and they quickly receive clot dissolving medicines, and they are immediately sent to the catheterization laboratory where a skilled cardiologist can open the blockage with a balloon angioplasty, and then a stent is inserted to open blood flow to the heart muscle, the process is a miracle. That's a long list of 'ifs.' However, if all this happens in perfect time, it's a great thing for a patient. Why? Well, if all this happens in perfect time, the heart muscle will not die and turn into scar tissue—which can cause countless problems down the road."

The results of angioplasty and stenting in the face of acute heart attack are dramatic. Obviously, if the condition is that dangerous, the whole process is absolutely necessary. And, it shows how far medicine has come, at least when we're discussing life saving processes.

"It is a life-saving miracle," says Dr. Lundell. "To watch an artery open, and see the blood begin to flow, and the heart muscle begin to pump again, would have been considered an impossible miracle not too long ago. It's amazing. The chance to dramatically alter the course of a heart attack, to save the heart muscle, to prevent disability and death is the reason the cardiologist will get up in the middle of the night—to save your life. My only wish is that it didn't have to happen in the first place—heart disease is curable long before we get to this point."

It's dangerous. It's dramatic. And, it's extremely costly. The current worldwide market for coronary stents is estimated at $5 billion. This market, and the demand for better results, drives medical companies to produce these items in mass quantity and spend huge amounts of money on research, development and promotion.

"The fascination with the latest technology and a desire to be the first on your block with a new tool has taken cardiologists away from curing heart disease," says Dr. Lundell. "Now, they're simply focused on performing a procedure not treating the disease, just like I did for many years. And, I think it's perfectly natural to attempt to solve an immediate problem. We still need those drastic measures in place. But, I'd like to see a change in the thought process—where we could refocus on the root cause of the disease. Sadly, that focus is difficult because nobody gets paid for it."

"But, I've been just as guilty as the rest," Dr. Lundell continues. "I was one of the founding partners of what is now known as Banner Baywood Heart Hospital. I had my office on the fifth floor and performed surgery on the third floor. And, I took care of critical patients in the ICU on the fourth floor. It is a beautiful building and a world-class facility. Nevertheless, the place is a monument to sickness—not to health. The physicians, nurses, administrators and other employees don't sit around hoping for good health in the population. All of our jobs were dependant on your bad health—not your good health. There's no incentive in the entire system to promote good health. An orthopedic surgeon doesn't sit around hoping you don't break your arm. Of course, he or she isn't hoping you break a bone, but without your ill fortune, they wouldn't have a job. They wouldn't be able to support their family or pay their mortgage. There is actually a joke where one doctor says to another, 'What you are doing today?' The other doctor replies, 'Just taking money from sick people.' That's sad."

It is sad. And, it's all too common.

How common is stenting? Following diagnostic cardiac catheterization, stenting is the most common procedure performed on the human heart. An estimated 1,000,000 of these procedures were performed in the United States in 2006, with an average cost of $38,203.

Statins

Here's another subject that has almost been discussed to a point of exhaustion—statin drugs. You can't watch television or read a magazine without seeing an advertisement for statins.

Do statins work? And, how well do they work compared to surgery or angioplasty?

"With surgery and angioplasty, the results are clear," says Dr. Lundell. "Complication, heart attack, death, and heart function are all easy to measure. Medical treatment on the other hand, in spite of the progress, has relatively few studies. In the 1970s, the available treatments were nitrates and a couple of diuretics. Since then, we have beta-blockers, calcium channel blockers, long-acting nitrates, ace inhibitors, and statins. Of all these medications, the only drugs studied vigorously are statins."

Statins aren't just studied vigorously, they're also marketed vigorously. Last year, the sales of Lipitor®, the statin made by Pfizer, reached $12.5 billion—making it the largest selling drug in the world.

"Obviously, the cholesterol theory on heart disease opened the doors of capitalism," says Dr. Lundell. "Anyone who could reduce cholesterol by creating a simple pill was bound to make money. But, you asked if they work. The first medications available blocked the absorption of cholesterol from the intestine. Those initial drugs were poorly tolerated and only mildly effective—due to the fact that approximately 80% of the cholesterol in our blood is manufactured by our liver. Other researchers approached the cholesterol issue by developing medications to block the production of cholesterol. This class of drugs is called statins. They exert their lipid-lowering effect by blocking an enzyme that's involved in the early stages of the production of cholesterol. Statins also block the production of many other important compounds, which derive during the production of cholesterol."

"I don't want to engage in an extensive search and critique of the volumes of medical literature relating to statins and cholesterol," adds Lundell. "There is a ton of medical literature written on both sides of the debate—whether they work or don't work, and why. However, while I am by no means a world authority on statins, I would like to offer the simple facts so you—along with your doctor—can make an informed decision as to whether or not statins would be a benefit to your health."

What does the current statin research prove?
* Statins *do* modestly lower blood cholesterol levels.

* Statins *do* modestly lower heart attack rates in middle-aged men with known coronary artery disease.

- Statins *do not* reduce mortality or heart attack rates in women.

- Statins *do not* lower mortality rates in men who have not been diagnosed with heart disease.

"There is research that shows very promising benefits of statin medications," says Dr. Lundell. "However, the benefits of statins may not be what you think. The benefits start long before there is a reduction in cholesterol levels."

Dr. Lundell says that statins have beneficial effects that are independent of lowering your cholesterol. "Statins can improve endothelial function. They have anti-clotting effects. They have positive antioxidant benefits. They may reduce the risk of plaque rupture. And, they've been shown to have anti-inflammatory effects."

Did he say, "Anti-inflammatory effects?"

"Statins seem to inhibit the artery wall from creating the Velcro-effect we discussed earlier," says Dr. Lundell. "They've also been shown to reduce C-reactive protein levels which are a key marker of inflammation. Yes, they have benefits. I wonder how long it will take before they are marketed differently—to reveal the true benefits. And, I know that many people reading this will ask if I recommend statins. And, I won't take sides. I will say this. Even though statins show many benefits, there are other ways of achieving the same health benefits—and the other options are definitely friendlier on your metabolism and your pocketbook."

Okay, so some aggressive measures may be necessary in the fight against heart disease. It's comforting to know that if an emergency situation arises, medicine has definitely advanced to the point where your odds of surviving a heart attack look a lot more promising today than they did just a few years ago.

"I support the fine doctors who perform miracles in dire situations," says Dr. Lundell. "But, we're talking about human life here. Yes, it's important to save lives. What about the cost of losing your quality of life? What about the physical toll, the loss of work, and the emotional toll some of these aggressive measures can have on your life? And, if the quality of your life is hard to measure, in terms of value, let's look at this whole picture as if it were a credit card commercial. Bypass surgery—$83,919. Cardiac Cath. with stent—$63,096. Statins and other meds—$250 per month. Getting healthy and staying healthy—priceless."

That's an ad campaign that works. However, there's one possible exception that might even make it more powerful. Maybe instead of using the word priceless, we should use the word free. Decisions cost nothing. And, by making the right decisions, we all might be able to use the word free a little more often—disease free, drug free, and surgery free.

Feel free to remove yourself from the list of statistics—all it takes is a simple decision to change your perspective. ⚕

Blazing Biology: The Perfect Firestorm

BY NOW, YOU'VE PROBABLY NOTICED the fact that every chapter in this book ends by granting you the power to initiate change. You have control.

By now, you've also read gobs of information. And, you're probably getting anxious to find out how all of this fits into one plan of action—one simple solution.

And, by now you're most likely beginning to understand the correlation between everything that has been discussed—it's one full circle where every action has a reaction, and every cell is connected.

By now, you're wondering, "what now?"

"Lives will be saved, one at a time," says Dr. Lundell. "At this point, we cannot fight this epidemic on a large scale. We know the real cause of heart disease. We know how the disease became an epidemic. The only thing we're missing is a response. And, I'll tell you right now that training and hiring more heart surgeons isn't the answer. I may have performed over five thousand surgeries, but that is just the top of the tip of the iceberg. The cure to this disease resides in each of us taking responsibility for ourselves."

Responsibility? Nobody likes that word. It means there's work involved. Nevertheless, we only have a few options to save ourselves.

Are you part of a growing epidemic?
Or, are you part of the cure?

Let's face it; the information you've learned up to this point has obviously communicated that no matter how many studies are conducted, how many recommendations are made, or how much money is thrown at the government to continue chasing the low-fat and low-cholesterol theory, you still have choices. You can choose what you eat. You can choose which information you want to incorporate into your lifestyle. The choices are still yours.

Is choice a responsibility? Or, is it an opportunity?

"We all have choices to make," says Lundell. "The only thing we cannot choose is how the current dietary recommendations affect our health. If you choose the low-fat and low-cholesterol diet, consequences will arise. Again, that brings us back to the facts. Your biology doesn't make choices—it simply responds to your choices."

So, how does your biology respond to the low-fat and low-cholesterol diet?

We already know how our nation has responded—low-fat has made us fatter and less healthy. And, although many of us could look back at the past 15 years and simply blame our current belt size on age or lack of exercise, how do we know that we're not really part of the epidemic—a mere result of a massive test theory without any scientific backing?

And, after all this, you're probably still thinking about the information from the last few chapters and wondering, what does fat have to do with inflammation? And, why does this chapter have such a goofy title?

What is a firestorm?

"The word inflammation means fire inside," says Lundell. "That's what is happening inside our body as we become a statistic of an epidemic. We're burning up from inflammation. The low-fat and low-cholesterol diet—along with other lifestyle choices—has created the perfect firestorm."

Huh? First we had a battlefield and now it's a firestorm? Inside our body?

Fire is created by combining heat, air, and fuel. If you remove anything from that list, the fire will be snuffed—it can no longer burn. When you apply that theory to the heart disease epidemic, it's easy to see a blaze within our bodies—fueled by a low-fat/high-carbohydrate diet, sparked by our own genetic biology, given life by physical inactivity, and burning out of control.

"We are all a product of our genetics, plus our environment," says Dr. Lundell. "And, when you really observe our genetic biology and how it responds to the environment, you can see where this thing has gone haywire—it's just like a massive fire."

So, imagine a log that you would use to create a fire. It's wood. That's easy enough. But, now consider the type of wood, the age of the wood, and the condition of the wood. All these variables could effect how that log burns. Will it burn quickly? Will it burn hot with a raging flame?

When it comes to our bodies, and how our genetics will react to our environment, who really knows how we'll respond to the inflammation fire? Aren't we like the piece of wood? Isn't every one of us different?

"We know how our bodies will respond," says Dr. Lundell. "We're the first generation with the capability to examine our DNA as humans and observe changes over time. All of us will be slightly different genetically. Obviously, our genetic history will play a role. However, we're all basically the same when it comes to the body's biological systems. All of our bodies will respond the same way to environmental changes—it's just a question of degrees."

Basically, Dr. Lundell is saying that all wood will burn if you set it on fire. Some will burn hotter, or faster, or even more easily. But, it all burns. And, the burning process is biologically the same.

"Our genome has not changed in the last 10,000 years," says Dr. Lundell. "Our bodies respond the same way now as they did way back then. They've been responding the same way since before the agricultural revolution. On the other hand, our environment has changed drastically even in just the past 20 years—both our diet and our activity level. And, that's a good thing. If our environment is the only thing that has changed, it means we can change it back."

Change our environment? What on earth does that mean?

Sure, we all know that our ancestors were required to exert themselves on a daily basis to secure their food, water and shelter. They were hunters and gatherers, walking or running five to ten miles a day. They had to track animals—even chase them through the woods with simple tools like spears. And, if they killed an animal, think of how much more exhausting it must have been just to get that animal back home. That's real work. And, if they couldn't slay a great piece of meat for dinner, they foraged for food like fruits and nuts—lifting, climbing, and doing whatever else it took to simply survive.

For us, modern technology has made physical exertion optional. In fact, achieving adequate physical activity is now a burden—simply because we can live our entire lives without exerting ourselves whatsoever. When do we find time to exercise? When do we find time to consider healthy living? Our environments are now exactly the opposite of our ancestors.

"Any living organism thrives best in the environment and on the diet to which it has genetically adapted," says Lundell. "This is a fundamental axiom of biology. So, all of a sudden the hunters and gatherers realized they had options. That's when they began using agricultural means to provide food. And, that made sense. It's difficult to establish societies and build communities if you're always following a herd of buffalo. Farming seemed to be a better way."

There's no doubt that farming was a revolutionary step. But, if a living organism changes its diet overnight, what happens? And, what if that farmer now sits on a tractor for ten hours a day instead of foraging for food, or hunting? All of sudden, our species is living a lifestyle that doesn't correlate with its own biological needs. So, what happens?

Consider even minor changes in your daily regime, like taking a vacation where you eat foods that your system isn't accustomed to consuming. We've all done that before—and we can spend a week feeling ill. Oops, there you are in paradise, lunged over a toilet regurgitating last night's seafood special. That's happened to most of us at some point. Eating foods that your body isn't accustomed to can create painful havoc.

Now, consider a change that is opposite of what our biology has grown accustomed to for thousands of years. We're no longer talking about a week-long case of nausea and upset stomach—we could spend the next thousand years getting ill—and it's possible that we will, unless we make a change.

"Today, in our nation, it's total chaos," says Lundell. "History has shown us that when hunters and gatherers switched to an agricultural based diet, they became substantially shorter, their general health deteriorated, they had shorter life spans, higher childhood mortality and higher incidence of all sorts of diseases. Now, I don't want to go back to those times, but a study of the differences in our dietary environment may help us adapt and avoid so-called diseases of convenience."

Current Health C.H.A.O.S. in America

C - Coronary disease
H - Hypertension
A - Adult onset Diabetes
O - Obesity
S - Stroke

The dietary recommendations made by the USDA food pyramid are as distant from what we are genetically designed to consume as the space shuttle is to Paleolithic man. Watching our nation suffer by this new regime of dietary guidelines is like watching a bad movie from the 80s where a caveman is revived to deal with modern society—sooner or later the change destroys him.

We're not living in caves. We know what's going on in the world. Don't we?

Who hasn't heard of the low-carb diet craze? Raise your hand.

When carbohydrates are mentioned, you most likely think of other popular diet fads—where carbohydrates are reduced or almost even eliminated from a diet. Do those diets work? Are they healthy? And what do carbohydrates have in common with heart disease?

"These low carbohydrate diets did work," says Dr. Lundell. "But, let's not get confused with some overnight weight loss plan and healthy living. Our country is so fixated on losing weight that sometimes we miss the big picture. Let's look to the facts. Let's look at biology. Let's look beyond simple weight loss. Let's talk about health."

Okay. What's next? Is he going to tell us something we didn't already know? The Zone and Atkins diets became the rage a few years back. We all know that. And, most of us have experimented with those diets. Then, public consensus stepped in and cried foul—these diets can't be healthy because there's that little food pyramid that says 9-11 servings of grains and cereals per day. Once again, our nation rests its faith in the system. There's no possible way that a concept that challenges the norm can be healthy. Or, can it?

"The foundation of the USDA food pyramid consists of refined grains and sugars," says Dr. Lundell. "But, there were no refined grains in our ancient diet. The closest thing to refined sugar was honey—and that was only when it could be found in season. Our ancestors didn't eat this stuff—none of it. If sugar is so necessary in our diets how did our ancestors survive?"

That's a good question. But, the solution can't be found in a box of crackers. Even if we eliminate our snacking of carbohydrates, we have other issues—we can choose not to eat grains, but our livestock can't choose their meals. And, if you've had the chance to see what you're last Thanksgiving turkey was fed, you might be feeling a bit queasy right about now.

"Our livestock is fat too," says Dr. Lundell. "The meat we consume today—cattle, poultry, pork, and even fish—are now grain fed. A few years ago, I was in a cattle feedlot where the cattle were fattened on the scraps of potatoes from a French fry factory. So, I guess the burger and fries are really the same thing. That's scary. Our meat may be less healthy than we are."

But, what's the big deal? Meat is meat, right? Although, it's not too appealing to consider the fact that our meat could be less healthy than we are. And, why the big fuss about carbohydrates anyway? Don't we need carbohydrates for energy? Why are carbohydrates so evil?

"We do need carbohydrates for energy," says Lundell. "But, where are we expending this extra energy? The low-fat high-carbohydrate diet causes us to have elevated blood glucose, which leads to increased production of insulin, which leads to fat storage, which leads to obesity, which leads to increased production by fat cells of inflammatory chemicals. And, elevated glucose and insulin play key roles in starting the inflammatory process."

Yikes. That was a list of biological reactions that isn't very pleasant. And, that same list holds true for many of the meat products we eat. So, basically the carbohydrates aren't good, the meat is no longer good, and even the fats we once consumed are now engineered to be worse. We'll touch on that topic in just a bit.

We already know that every action has a reaction. So, how are our poor bodies—that were once genetically accustomed to hunting and gathering—reacting to this new of form diet?

"We're dying," says Lundell. "That's it."

Right now is where everything you've learned so far in this book leads right back to where we started—your body fighting a battle against inflammation.

"The inflammatory chemicals (cytokines) created through the string of biological processes—insulin production, fat storage, and obesity—will cause the inside of our arteries to become sticky like Velcro as we have previously discussed," says Lundell. "The high blood sugar and high insulin levels cause changes in the low-density lipoprotein (LDL) which the white cells (remember those macrophages, the really aggressive immune system warriors), then attempt to destroy, because they think it's a foreign substance. Watch out, you're in the middle of a blazing fire."

Wow! That's a lot to digest. A few extra carbohydrates and suddenly we're dying?

Well, if this isn't irony, what is? If our ancestors never consumed refined sugars, wouldn't the body naturally consider them a foreign substance? And, if our ancestors were burning off excess energy (carbohydrates) by hunting and gathering, wouldn't elevated insulin and excess fat storage be considered foreign?

"Our genetics aren't equipped to deal with refined sugars," says Lundell. "The high sugar and high insulin levels in the blood disturb or agitate the lining of the blood cells by themselves. Of course our natural defense system will fight back. All of sudden, we're a huge battleground of inflammation. Grain based diets also overload our system with omega 6 free fatty acids. These omega 6 fats are pro-inflammatory. They make every cell membrane abnormally stiff."

Starch is for shirts, not for arteries.

Is eating a low carbohydrate diet the big secret to reducing inflammation?

"Starch is for shirts, not for arteries," says Lundell. "Starch and refined sugars do a lot more damage than we ever imagined. Refined carbohydrates cause our bodies to produce high levels of insulin from our pancreas. Gradually, the cells become resistant to insulin. This is type II diabetes. The cells become less sensitive because of the consistently high levels of insulin, and because the cell walls have become abnormally stiff, due to an overload of omega 6 free fatty acids."

Do you see the vicious circle yet? Every time we consume more sugars than our bodies use, we create a cycle of internal terror. And, that's because our bodies are designed to eliminate the toxic substances.

"The cycle will continue even after a person stops consuming refined carbohydrates," says Dr. Lundell. "Overloaded fat cells will also produce a substance called resistin, which makes the cells even less responsive to insulin. So, the body will attempt to produce even more insulin to drive the sugar into the cells. This is what the body is supposed to do—and it's directly correlated to coronary artery disease."

Oh, and if you're still curious about how cholesterol plays into this scenario—how it became the indicator of heart disease—this is where it pops into the picture.

"LDL is changed in this environment, to become abnormal," says Lundell. "This is where all those studies were finding deposits of cholesterol in the artery wall. And, this is the scientific evidence that cholesterol deposits are actually created by low-fat and low-cholesterol dietary habits—not by consuming dietary cholesterol."

So, there you are, nibbling away at your big box of low-fat crackers while your body is becoming a blaze of the perfect firestorm. Inflammatory cytokines are bouncing around your body trying to fight battles in parts of your body that you never even knew existed. Shucks, there's another battle in your left pinky toe, one in your abdomen, and one up in the back corner of your skull. Inflammation is everywhere.

That's just the simple version—cytokines are defending their homeland in every nook and cranny of your body. What's the complicated version? This is when Dr. Lundell throws out some words that may seem like tongue twisters. However, if you learn these words you'll be surprised by how often they'll soon be mentioned in the mass media—they are about to become common, everyday language of the American public.

"The facts are just beginning to be revealed," says Lundell. "Soon, everyone will start hearing about words like *interleukin 6* and *tumor necrosis factor alpha*. These are inflammatory chemicals that cause the liver to produce *C-reactive protein*. C-reactive protein is the easily measured marker of inflammation in the blood. And, very soon it will become one of the most publicly visible terms used in the media when they discuss health, longevity, wellness, and disease. Soon every physical examination will test for C-reactive protein. It will become a primary indicator of many diseases—including cancer, Alzheimer's, heart disease, diabetes, and stroke. Watch for it. And remember, you knew about it before anyone else."

Why should you pay attention to C- reactive protein?

Well, because it's the primary marker for how much inflammation that exists in our bodies—it's the proof, the measuring stick, and the meter. It's how we can keep score in the war against inflammation.

Recent research has demonstrated that C- reactive protein binds with leptin. Leptin is the hormone that is produced by fat cells which tells our bodies to stop eating. And when C- reactive protein binds with leptin, our brains no longer recognize leptin. That means we'll continue to eat, and eat, and eat.

"It becomes a vicious cycle," says Lundell. "Once the cycle starts, that choice we had early on at the grocery store becomes less of a choice—now it's an impulse to feed the fire. It starts with excess simple carbohydrates, and the wrong kind of fats. It creates inflammation, obesity, unresponsive cells, and interruption of normal physiological control mechanisms—more eating, less satisfaction, and one huge health crisis. The epidemic in America isn't just heart disease. We have a diabetes epidemic, an obesity epidemic and a myriad of other diseases that are caused by this cycle of inflammation, like hypertension, Alzheimer's, kidney failure, limb loss, infertility, arthritis and the list goes on."

Just for the sake of reiteration—and to drill this point into our skulls when we take the advice of public consensus, or a misguided food label, or feel the sudden urge to gobble up a plate of cup cakes—remember, our cells are all living and they are all connected. All the diseases listed earlier are fueled by the same thing—starches and sugar. They're actually all very similar.

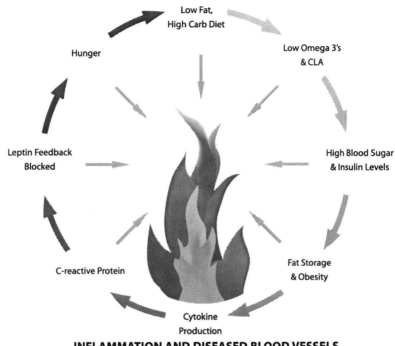

INFLAMMATION AND DISEASED BLOOD VESSELS

"I call this vicious cycle, the perfect firestorm," says Lundell. "It is self perpetuating, it builds on itself, and it slowly then rapidly destroys everything around it—creating all sorts of diseases. I have seen this storm. I have touched this storm. I have battled this storm. Now, I want to give you the tools to stop it from occurring, stop it before it takes your life or simply steals your health. You can repair the damage that has occurred."

Wait a second. If all the diseases are similar, wouldn't it make sense that they all can be prevented and even cured through the same biological processes?

Yes. Good health and bad health flows through the same vessels.

That's the good news. The same pathways that carry dangerous things throughout our bodies are also the pathways of recovery. Remember, the arteries control our circulation, both how much blood flows, and exactly where it is distributed. If the arteries become abnormal because of inflammation, the whole body becomes abnormal as well. If the arteries become healthy, so will the body.

Here's an easy way to think about it. It's much like our modern transportation system—freeways, major streets, minor streets, and alleys. Goods and services are delivered, and waste products are taken away, all on the same roads. Now, if some of the traffic signals are disrupted—like if a stoplight goes on the blink—things won't get properly delivered, garbage won't be properly removed, and normal life gets disrupted.

Now, if a major intersection is out of commission, we could take a detour. We all know that a detour isn't the path of least resistance, and it can be a pain in the neck. Nevertheless, our bodies will adapt to detours, and do the best they can to keep traffic flowing—detour or no detour.

But, just because traffic is flowing, doesn't mean there isn't a detour. And, just because blood continues to flow, doesn't mean there isn't a major health problem waiting in the alley to steal your life.

"If an artery is slowly becoming blocked, small collateral vessels will open up to take the flow," says Dr. Lundell. "It's not normal flow, but it is still flow—and it still ensures survival. It is amazing to see plugged arteries—jammed with disgusting slimy yellow junk—and the person can still be semi-functional. The reason I bring this up—the blood flow, and how the body will find alternate paths to survive—is simply to illustrate that many people walking around today are time bombs. And, they have no clue that they're in extreme danger. You don't have to be overweight to have heart disease. The fatty streaks happen internally even in very thin people. You don't even need to have insulin levels that are out of control or unstable. In fact, you don't need any of the symptoms discussed to be walking on the edge of death."

The edge of death? That's not a comforting thought. You might be reviewing your daily caloric intake of carbohydrates right about now— the pancakes for breakfast, the hoagie for lunch and that scrumptious pasta dish for dinner. All of these foods are being converted to sugar when they hit your bloodstream, creating a massive battle inside your body—a vicious circle that could spiral out of control.

Scary huh? So, what are you eating? What is your family eating?

To start, we consume a lot of sugar. Before 1900, sugar was a luxury item. The average American consumed less than 10 pounds per year. Today, it is estimated that we consume about 170 pounds of sugar per year.

And, that's refined sugar going into our mouths, not the sugars our body produces from consuming carbohydrates.

Following World War II, mechanized farming began producing abundant supplies of grain at relatively low cost. Advances in the production and distribution of commercial bakery products and pastas made refined wheat products, a staple of our diet. Prepackaged breads, cookies and other ready-to-eat products gained wide public acceptance. The low-fat dogma greatly increased the sugar and starch content of these foods and the amount of grains we consumed. Hey, if the box says it's low-fat, we could consume more, right? Let's be honest; our current diet has become predominantly refined grains and sugars.

And, if that's not bad enough, we even changed our fats to become less healthy.

For most of the 1900s, the major sources of dietary fat were butter, lard, coconut and olive oil. However, our nation's irrational fear of fat stimulated the development of new sources of edible fats and oil—created primarily from vegetable seeds. These new fats and oils needed to undergo a process called hydrogenation to keep them from becoming rancid in storage and prevent smoking during cooking.

Hydrogenation is simply the process of heating oil to a high temperature, and then bubbling hydrogen through the product in the presence of a catalyst—nickel. That's more than you probably care to know, but the result is something that cannot be overlooked.

When these new hydrogenated fats and oils are used in baked goods, the shelf life significantly increases and the product can be listed as a low-fat substitute.

Unfortunately, these products are the Frankenstein of foods. The hydrogenation process creates trans-fats and destroys essential free fatty acids that are required for human life and health. How do you think our hunter and gatherer biology responds to synthetic gunk? Can anybody say foreign substance?

Today, it is estimated that Americans consume an average of 40 pounds a year of this synthetic Frankenstein fat, which never in our history was part of the human diet. What's that doing to our bodies?

Is it merely a coincidence that heart disease began to increase after the invention of Crisco in 1912—the first hydrogenated oil/trans fat to be consumed by humans?

"It's a scary situation," says Dr. Lundell. "All foods are composed of the same few basic nutrients—proteins, carbohydrates, fats and other lipids, vitamins, and minerals. The nutritional quality of a diet is thus dependent on what foods are selected to be in that diet. As a nation, we've made the wrong choices. But, that's good. That means that we can still make the right choices. And, why not make the right choices? If a diet contributes to, or causes a chronic disease that could ultimately cause disability and death, why not choose foods that promote health?"

Dr. Lundell may have been too kind in his word choices in that last statement. Statistically, unless you die of a tragic accident, one of the diseases mentioned in this chapter will become your fate—heart disease, diabetes, stroke, Alzheimer's, obesity, or some other disease caused by poor food choices.

If you step into the street without looking both ways, and get smacked by a bus, it's your fault. If you walk into a grocery store and buy foods without looking at healthier options, well, it's your own fault.

"This is life or death," says Lundell. "This is your life, or your mother's life, or your child's life. And, it's not just about dying. Living with advanced heart disease or obesity or Alzheimer's isn't a good quality of life. The low-fat and low-cholesterol dogma is now so ingrained, and so supported by such a wide variety of industries, government agencies, drug makers, with such powerful economic interests, that it will be very difficult to change. But, we don't have to change it. We simply need to make choices for our own lives. That's where we get power."

Are you ready to take control?

You've learned a lot. You've probably questioned your own perspectives on health. You've probably questioned the decisions you make on a daily basis. And, hopefully the information has been disturbing enough, disgusting enough, and clear enough to make you realize that you can challenge public consensus. You can overcome a national epidemic. And, you're ready to battle the firestorm that is inflaming your body.

Your body isn't a machine with separate parts. Your life isn't dependant on misguided assumptions. And, your world isn't flat.

"Neither you nor I are forced to be slaves to consensus," says Dr. Lundell. We wouldn't be here in America if Christopher Columbus believed the world was flat. I wouldn't be here telling you how to cure heart disease if I hadn't challenged my own career—a career focused on fixing something only after it has been broken. Ironically, we're still fixing something that's broken—it's not our hearts, it's our system of beliefs. We don't have to continue to take dietary advice that is slowly killing us. I don't have to, and you don't have to."

What can you do?

"Keep reading," says Lundell. "We're just getting to the good stuff—

squashing the firestorm, eliminating disease, and even losing a few pounds in the process. This is where the fun starts—and the rest of your healthy life." ⊬

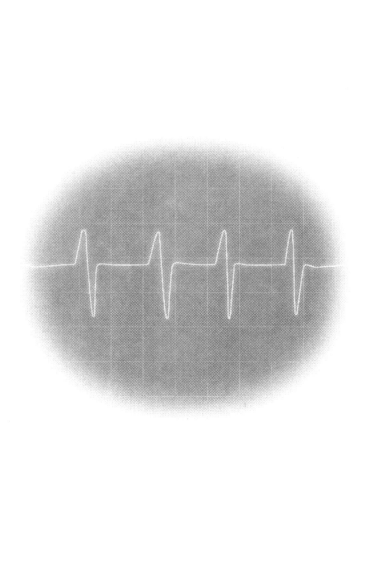

Fighting the Fire
of Inflamation

WHAT HAPPENS WHEN A FIRE starts?

When a building or structure is engulfed by flames, the sirens blare, the hoses roll out, the ladders go up, and oodles of brave firemen swarm the premises to save lives and extinguish the blaze. They douse the building with water and fire-retardant chemicals, they attempt to suffocate the oxygen that keeps the fire breathing, and they remove any fuels that could potentially make the fire grow even more destructive.

A fire is an emergency. Response must happen immediately or people die.

But, what happens after a fire? What happens after all the damage has occurred?

After a fire has been extinguished, many people remain shocked, wondering how the fire started in the first place. And, most of the time, everybody reacts as if the fire started instantaneously—by some unruly kid playing with matches, a building tenant falling asleep with a cigarette, or an overzealous chef who accidentally spawns a grease fire.

Although these type of things are often the cause of the fire, the reality is often a lot less dramatic—faulty wiring or electronics, heating units not properly used or installed or numerous other "boring" reasons. Ask any member of the fire department and they'll tell you horror stories of homeowners who stacked firewood on top of their wood burning stoves, or do-it-yourself contractors who installed lighting fixtures incorrectly.

After a fire is extinguished is when insurance companies arrive on the scene to determine exactly how the fire started—they want to know the cause. And, many times, when the cause of a fire is 'boring', the experts will say, "This fire could have been prevented a long time ago," or "This fire could have been smoldering for days before it ignited."

Sad but true, inflammation is much like a 'boring' fire. Inflammation smolders inside our bodies—never giving us any signs of the lurking dangers until disease, disability and disaster strike.

So, how do you get rid of the inflammation? How do you prevent the fire inside? And, if your fire is already blazing, how do you extinguish it before it burns us to the ground?

"With inflammation, we get to be the firemen," says Dr. Lundell. "We can prevent inflammation, and we can extinguish it. We can cure heart disease by putting out the fire."

Okay, so now that we've already consumed a tremendous amount of information—some of it being complex—you're probably wondering how difficult it is to manage your own fire so you can cure heart disease.

"First of all, we need to decide where the fire is," says Dr. Lundell. "In this particular case it's in our arteries. And, now that we all understand the mechanisms of arterial inflammation, we can determine the best fire extinguisher to apply, and what preventative measures to use, to stop inflammation in its tracks. Remember, this is about using the facts to our advantage. We cannot cure disease without the right diagnosis. But, we have the science to provide the correct diagnosis, which means we can apply the best treatment."

What are the causes of chronic low-grade inflammation? Can we eliminate those causes? And, if we cannot eliminate the causes, how can we reduce the damage and manage the danger?

Be warned. What you're about to read next, may sound familiar. At the beginning of this book we mentioned how a discussion focused on heart disease may sound like a broken record. You may look at the sub-headings below and assume that you know what is coming next. But, don't assume. That's how we ended up in this predicament in the first place! And, you might be surprised by the approach to these reoccurring topics—these are based on science, instead of public consensus.

Smoking

Unless you have been living in a time warp, you already know that smoking is bad for your health. But, why is bad for you? Is it the tar? Is it the smoke? Is it the nicotine?

"Cigarette smoking is dangerous to your heart because it causes arterial inflammation," says Dr. Lundell. "And, we won't even touch what kind of damage it does to your lungs. Just keep in mind that we're not a bunch of separate mechanical body parts. Every thing is connected. But, when it comes to the cardiovascular system, the chemicals from cigarette smoke directly damage the lining cells of the arteries—encouraging the white blood cells and any oxidized or damaged lipid to enter the medial layer of the artery."

Basically, when you take a drag, the smoke enters the lungs, gets passed into the blood stream, and gets passed throughout your entire cardiovascular system. And, from what we've learned about inflammation, the more the arterial walls are irritated, the more difficult it is for healing to take place. So, each cigarette adds insult to injury and impedes healing. Over time, your body's natural defense system goes haywire.

Hypertension

High blood pressure is also a common topic in the news. You may have already taken steps to reduce your blood pressure. But, why is high blood pressure so dangerous?

"High blood pressure puts stress on the vessels directly injuring the lining cells," says Dr. Lundell. "In reality, high blood pressure is much like smoking—this time, the pressure is irritating the lining and causing our bodies to respond with inflammation. High blood pressure is associated with high levels of angiotensin, a potent vasoconstrictor, which narrows the blood vessels and makes the pressure go up. Angiotensin also initiates the 'Velcro Effect' we spoke of earlier—appearing inside the blood vessel, so the inflammatory cascade gets started in multiple ways. It's also interesting that fat cells produce a precursor to angiotensin—a common side effect of obesity. Again, the body is all interconnected at the cellular level—one health problem can initiate another."

Oh, but wait. The circle doesn't stop there. Hypertension can also be the result of inflammation.

It causes inflammation and is a result of inflammation? Can it be?

Golly, it seems like we just can't win. When blood vessels stiffen as a result of inflammation, the vessel wall loses its ability to dilate. That means the vessel can no longer accommodate increased blood flow and, just like that, your blood pressure goes up. Again, it's a vicious circle of events that ultimately leads to destruction.

Elevated Blood Sugar

The association between diabetes and coronary artery disease has been known for some time. Type II diabetes is a disease caused by chronic over-consumption of simple carbohydrates. Remember those low-fat cookies? And, what about the 9 to 11 suggested servings of breads, grains and cereals in the food pyramid?

Over-consumption of simple carbohydrates results in chronic elevation of blood sugar and serum insulin. Basically, carbohydrates turn into sugar once they hit your blood stream.

"It becomes a vicious cycle," says Lundell. "Eat more sugar, produce more insulin, store more fat, experience excessive hunger, and eat more sugar. In the presence of chronic high sugar and insulin, the cells become less sensitive to insulin. Doctors will usually prescribe a medicine that'll help your pancreas make more insulin. There are also medications that make the cells more sensitive, or attempt to restore sensitivity. If worse comes to worse, they'll start the patient on insulin supplementation. That's when you know it's bad."

Again, it all comes back to inflammation. High blood sugar causes the lining cells of the arteries to be inflamed, changes LDL cholesterol, and causes sugar to be attached to a variety of proteins, which changes their normal function.

"This is why it's so important to understand the biology of inflammation," says Dr. Lundell. "High blood sugar in the arteries causes inflammation. Cytokines are elevated, the 'Velcro Effect' begins to form in the artery lining and arteriosclerosis begins. It's interesting that we focus so much on smoking and how it will harm people, but the focus on carbohydrates just isn't there. Type II diabetes has numerous consequences—it affects the very small blood vessels, which causes blindness, kidney failure and amputations."

Omega 6 Overload

What is omega 6? Where does it come from? And, why is it dangerous?

"With the substitution of animal fats in the Western diet with vegetable fats, we have become overloaded with omega 6 essential free fatty acids," says Lundell. "Omega 6 fatty acid is not inherently harmful in the right amounts. Omega 6 fatty acids tend to be metabolized into pro-inflammatory compounds—they promote inflammation. On the other hand, omega 3 essential free fatty acids tend to be metabolized into anti-inflammatory compounds—they help reduce inflammation. And, our diets are way off base when it comes to how much omega 6 we consume, and how little omega 3 we consume. According to the typical western diet, we're consuming a truckload of omega 6 and just a cup full of omega 3. Obviously the results will be detrimental. The current ratio in the American diet is about 20-to-1, omega 6 to omega 3. It should be somewhere between 4-to-1 and 1-to-1."

Omega 6 is found in vegetable oils, which are used in many of our modern cooking methods.

Population	Omega 6 Tissue Levels	Heart Attack deaths per 100,000
Greenland	30	20
Japanese	47	50
Mediterranean	58	90
American	78	200

Omega 3 Deficiency

Oh, c'mon! With our nation's tendency to over-indulgence, how can we be deficient in anything?

135

Diseases like rickets, beriberi and scurvy have basically vanished, yet 90% of Americans are deficient in omega 3. Is a deficiency still dangerous?

"The changes in our food supply have created a significant deficiency of omega 3 essential free fatty acids," says Dr. Lundell. "Why are they called essential? Well, because we cannot live without them. And, our bodies don't naturally create them, so they must be consumed as part of our diet. Some omega 3 can be obtained from green vegetables, nuts and seeds. However, the most beneficial source of omega 3 is fatty fish such as anchovies, sardines, mackerel, herring, trout, tuna and salmon."

Omega 3 essential free fatty acids are metabolized into anti-inflammatory compounds and combat the effect of omega 6 overload.

Trans-Fats

Remember the previous discussion on hydrogenation? Trans-fats are created by taking vegetable oil, heating it to a high temperature, and then bubbling hydrogen through it using nickel as a catalyst. Food manufacturers use the hydrogenation process to increase the product's shelf life and reduce smoke during the cooking process. Trans-fats are commonly found in commercial baked goods, restaurant cooking, deep-frying, and most vegetable oils.

"Trans-fats are an artificial compound, never before present in the human diet, and they wreak havoc on the human body," says Dr. Lundell. "These fats are nasty. Trans-fats interfere with the metabolism of omega 3—so even if we were getting enough omega 3 in our diet, we may not receive the anti-inflammatory benefits. Trans-fats have also been shown to increase C reactive protein, the marker for chronic low-grade inflammation."

Stress

Raise your hand and take a deep breath if you're feeling a little stress just from reading about stress. Perfect, now you need to be stressed about stress? Why and how can stress lead to inflammation?

"Our bodies are genetically programmed to handle acute stress without difficulty," says Dr. Lundell. "But, stress is another built-in biological defense mechanism of the body. And, just like the rest of our genetic programming, it hasn't changed. The only thing that has changed is our environment. When we encounter a stressful situation, our adrenal glands pour adrenaline into our system. This increases our heart rate, moves blood away from the intestines, and sends it toward the muscles. This is the so-called 'fight or flight' reaction. Our bodies prepare us to either fight an enemy or flee. However, we're not programmed for the chronic and consistent stress many of experience in the modern world. Some stresses are unavoidable, and some are self-inflicted. Chronic stress has been shown to increase the levels of cytokines in our blood—initiating the Velcro Effect, which attracts white blood cells, and again places us in a state of constant inflammation. The big question is: where is the inflammation? And the only answer I can provide is: just keep in mind that every cell is connected. It could show up anywhere."

Obesity

Look around. Most of us need to shed a few pounds. That's not news. And, although the definition of obesity can vary, the result of excess body weight has drastic results.

"Excess body weight, especially the fat we carry around our waists has been clearly demonstrated to release pro inflammatory cytokines into the circulation," says Dr. Lundell. "As you know, these cytokines are the early triggers of inflammation. As we discussed earlier, obesity is both a cause and a result of inflammation."

He continues, "It seems odd at first, but when you really think about it, it makes perfect sense. I couldn't help asking, 'why are my fat cells trying to poison me?' Why would my own body do something harmful? It doesn't seem fair until we realize that we have been poisoning our fat cells with trans fats, excess sugar and the wrong kind of fats. Fat cells are living organisms too. I'm not suggesting that they are seeking revenge on us, or that it's a bad case of karma, but that scientifically it makes sense. If we give our cells poison to work with, we're bound to get poisoned in return."

Vitamin Deficiency/Homocysteine

While the obvious vitamin deficiency diseases such as scurvy, beriberi, rickets and neural tube defects have been eliminated by vitamin fortified foods, supplements, and education, research is now showing that there are more subtle deficiencies that, over time, can have dangerous consequences on our health.

"Today, we understand and recognize the necessity of specific vitamins, and the role they play in our overall health," says Dr. Lundell. "In fact, our knowledge and ability to accurately measure vitamin and mineral levels within the body, has given a great insight into helping the body fight disease naturally. For example, sub-optimal levels of folic acid, vitamin B6 and B12 are known risk factors for heart disease, breast and colon cancer, Alzheimer's disease, reduced mental acuity and congenital neural tube defects. Deficiency in these B vitamins within the body causes an abnormal amount of homocysteine to circulate in our blood. High levels of homocysteine directly irritates the lining all our blood vessels, triggering the inflammatory process that causes arteriosclerosis."

Low levels of the antioxidant vitamins, A, C, and E are also associated with many chronic diseases in addition to heart disease.

Grab your extinguishers. We're about to douse the flames.

Now we know the causes of the fire. How do we fight it?

You wouldn't swat a fly on your knee with a sledgehammer because the side effects would be so dangerous and painful. You also wouldn't call in a fire truck to extinguish a small grease fire that is contained in a pan. So, how aggressive should we be fighting our internal fire?

"We don't need to treat chronic low-grade inflammation of the arteries with extremely powerful drugs," says Dr. Lundell. "We've seen what happens when we get overly aggressive. Vioxx, Celebrex and Bextra are three extremely powerful anti-inflammatory medications that had the unfortunate side effect of causing heart attacks. That kind of power wasn't necessary. And, besides, are we creating health by using these power-packed solutions, or are we back to square one? Are these highly aggressive drugs just a bandage that covers up why we have the inflammation in the first place?"

Hold on! Dr. Lundell, we're fighting a fire! Shouldn't we be as aggressive as possible?

"The only way to cure a disease is to treat it biologically—not just medicate it," says Dr. Lundell. "The most powerful anti-inflammatory substances are steroids. And, the most well known steroid is a medication called Prednisone—a synthetic corticosteroid that is similar to the natural steroids made in our adrenal glands. Prednisone not only suppresses inflammation, but also suppresses immunity."

Suppressing immunity isn't good. That could just lead to increased inflammation by allowing more infection into our body—more demons to call out more natural defenses which lead to continued inflammation.

If immunity is suppressed too much, even common invaders can overwhelm us—even kill us. Examples are: HIV and aids patients dying from otherwise trivial organisms, and transplant patients who die from the slightest infection.

"Prednisone—and similar anti-inflammatory medications—should be used in certain circumstances," says Lundell. "They should be used in the treatment of severe arthritis, allergic reactions, asthma, inflammatory bowel disease, organ transplantation, and certain other replacement therapies when our adrenal glands might be in a weakened state or failing. The problem is that this type of medication suppresses our own production of natural steroids if it's taken more than seven days in a row. We're curing heart disease—it takes more than seven days. Plus, short-term side effects of Prednisone are high blood glucose and fluid retention. Long-term side effects include weight gain, osteoporosis, and glaucoma."

We don't want that! So, are anti-inflammatory drugs bad for us? They seem like the easiest solution—the quick fix.

"Pharmaceuticals are not bad if they're used correctly," says Lundell.

"A simple aspirin isn't bad at all."

But, why would we subject ourselves to possible side effects of drugs if we can reduce or eliminate inflammation, and ultimately cure disease by using natural methods. Keep in mind, the only way to cure a disease is to eliminate the cause—not just mask the symptoms. Which brings us back to the topic of aspirin—why are so many doctors recommending an aspirin a day? Is it for pain relief?

Aspirin is the oldest documented anti-inflammatory, which originally derived from the bark of a willow tree. Currently, Americans consume roughly 80 million aspirin tablets each day. But, even more interesting is the evolution of a common aspirin—from basic pain reliever to popular anti-inflammatory drug.

The discovery of aspirin began in 1895 when a young German chemist began researching salicylates, a naturally occurring group of chemicals found in a wide range of foods, herbs and spices. Salicylates had for centuries been used to relieve pain. However, the taste was bitter, and it often caused vomiting. After several years of work the German researcher combined salicylic acid with vinegar and found that the combination retained its pain relieving benefits, but eliminated the bad taste and vomiting.

Bingo! Aspirin was born. The company that young chemist was working for is now known as Bayer—likely the world's most recognized pharmaceutical brand.

However, even though aspirin was so widely used, it wasn't until the 1970's that scientists figured out exactly how aspirin works in our body. In fact, a British pharmacologist by the name of John Vane received the Nobel Prize in medicine for his revolutionary discovery in 1982—aspirin wasn't just pain relief, it reduced acute inflammation, which is the number one cause of pain.

"Aspirin is the most prominent member of a family of drugs called non-steroidal anti-inflammatory drugs, sometimes referred to more commonly as NSAIDS," says Dr. Lundell. "Other NSAIDS include ibuprofen, which have brand names like Aleve and Motrin. The newest members of the NSAIDS family are called COX 2 inhibitors such as Vioxx and Celebrex."

Those are all names we're quite familiar with—there's got to be a television commercial airing at any given moment promoting at least one of these drugs. But, these are painkillers. And, if pain is caused by inflammation, is there a chance that by biologically reducing acute inflammation within the body, we could also get rid of our common aches and pains?

"NSAIDS do what are bodies are supposed to do, if we were providing ourselves with everything we needed to reduce inflammation naturally," says Lundell. "All NSAID's act by inhibiting the enzyme cyclo-oxygenase (otherwise known as COX). This is an enzyme that converts arachidonic acid (sometimes referred to as AA) to prostaglandin 2 (abbreviated as PG2). Prostaglandins act as messenger molecules in the process of inflammation. There are three types of prostaglandins."

Okay, admittedly, these sound like big 'doctorish' words. Why do you need to know these gigantic words? Why are you twisting your brain and your tongue to pronounce prostaglandins?

"As the research about inflammation becomes more publicized, these words will become well known," says Dr. Lundell. "America is in for a big new surprise. I just hope for the sake of curing heart disease that the media storm comes sooner than later."

PG1, PG2, and PG3 are the three types of prostaglandins that will receive publicity. Why do we care about PG1, PG2, and PG3?

- PG1 reduces inflammation, inhibits blood clotting, dilates blood vessels, and helps the body recover by reducing pain, swelling, and redness.

- PG2 has the opposite effect. It encourages blood clotting, constricts blood vessels and increases inflammation. Just remember, PG2 is the bad one!

- PG3 has a mixture of functions in protecting the body from injury. One of its most important functions is to reduce the production of PG2.

There. Whew. Done. Had enough of the heavy medical terminology?

That's the basic explanation of NSAIDS. All the brand names you see on television and on the shelves at your local pharmacy are basically performing the same function of reducing inflammation—to different degrees, of course, depending on whether we're talking about over the counter or prescription medications. However aspirin is the only one that makes the blood platelets less sticky, which reduces blood clotting, and makes it even more beneficial.

Before all this gives you a headache, and you need to take aspirin, let's step back from the big words and review.

Immunity: The state of having sufficient biological defenses, to avoid infection, disease, or other biological invasion. This means having antibodies, white blood cells, and other means to recognize a biological invasion and call out the army to fight it.

Inflammation: The body's natural response when the immune system recognizes an invasion. The outcome in any particular invasion will be determined by the strength of the invader, the resilience of the tissue that it invades, and your body's specific response.

Generally, there are four possible outcomes of an inflammatory attack.

1. Resolution: The defeat of the invader and the return of the tissue to normal.

2. Scarring: Usually about 24 hours after an invasion occurs a wound healing response begins new blood vessels are formed to provide nutrients and connective tissue is formed. The most common place, we see this is after a skin laceration.

3. Abscess Formation: This most commonly occurs when the invader is a bacteria or a foreign body, like a sliver. The scar tissue surrounds the battlefield and contains it to a small area, which turns into pus.

4. Chronic Inflammation: If the injury continues, continued inflammation is the result. Chronic inflammation is dominated by white blood cells, called macrophages. Macrophages not only gobble up the invader, but they also produce chemicals in an attempt to destroy the invader. Some of these chemicals (cytokines) are designed to call for reinforcements. Remember

the inside of the blood vessel, turning to Velcro to attract more white cells.

"Heart disease is caused by chronic low-grade inflammation," says Dr. Lundell "I don't know if I can reiterate that simple statement enough. And, if we directly fight the causes of the fire within our body, we will cure heart disease. It's that simple."

Are you ready for the simple solutions—the extinguishers to fight the fire?

Fires are fought by dousing flames with water or fire-retardants. Fires are fought by removing any forms of fuel that can keep the fire burning. And, fires are fought by suffocating the dangerous environment—leaving an environment that is fire resistant.

Extinguisher #1— Douse the Fire

"The first thing we can do to reduce inflammation is consume more essential free fatty acids," says Dr. Lundell. "I cannot stress the importance of this enough. Essential free fatty acids are essential because our bodies don't produce them naturally—they must be obtained from our diet."

There are two groups, of the essential free fatty acids: omega 3 fatty acids, and omega 6 fatty acids. These fatty acids have numerous functions. First, they are structural components of every cell membrane— they ensure stability, flexibility and act as gatekeepers for the cell.

Second, they are converted into prostaglandins. The omega 3 fatty acids are converted into prostaglandin one (PG1) anti-inflammatory, and the omega 6 fatty acids are converted into prostaglandin 2 (PG2) pro-inflammatory.

Yes, you read that correctly. PG1 reduces inflammation. PG2 promotes inflammation

"Both are essential for survival," says Lundell. "The ratio of omega 6 to omega 3 is critically important in the function of every cell. Just like in your high school chemistry experiment. If you overload one chemical versus another you get an entirely different result—a dangerous result."

But, how do we know how to balance that ratio? As we discussed earlier, the typical American diet is significantly overloaded with omega 6 and significantly deficient in omega 3. How important is it to balance these free fatty acids?

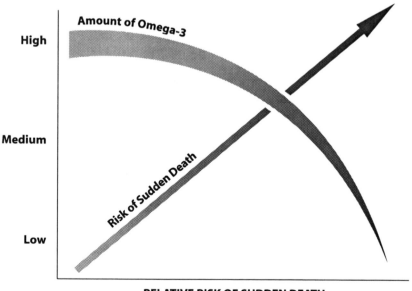

RELATIVE RISK OF SUDDEN DEATH
COMPARED TO RED BLOOD CELL OMEGA-3 LEVELS

"If you learn nothing else from this book, learn this," cautions Lundell. "Omega 3 free fatty acids act as targeted fire extinguishers against chronic inflammation. They are naturally powerful anti-inflammatory substances that have no adverse effects on acute inflammation or immunity. We need more omega 3 in our diet."

Targeted extinguishers? A better explanation might be a guided missile—with multiple laser-guided precision warheads. Unlike a broad carpet-bomb approach by suppressing all inflammatory activity, like Prednisone and, to a lesser extent, the Cox inhibitors, omega 3 specifically targets inflammation sites further down the inflammatory chain—inhibiting the activity of chronic inflammation without interfering with immunity or the body's ability to respond to an invader.

"Here we go back to the immunity battlefield," says Dr. Lundell. "Omega 3 reduces the effectiveness of the cytokines that cause the Velcro Effect. Remember, those little Velcro fingers grab the mono-cytes and hold them against the vessel wall. Omega 3 manages the monocytes—they kind of place them 'at ease' so they don't send out too many cytokines to call for reinforcements. Basically, omega 3 calms the battle so inflammation doesn't get out of control."

So, instead of calling out the warlords of inflammation, omega 3 calls out the coolers—the firefighters and the peacemakers. Remember, omega 3 competes with omega 6 to be converted to prostaglandins, which creates more anti-inflammatory prostaglandins.

"Omega 3 affects the cell wall of every cell in our body," says Lundell. "I'd love to reveal all the research we have that demonstrates the anti-inflammatory benefits of omega 3. But, it's impossible in this book to review the over 4500 articles of medical literature. Just be aware that all of the articles show the beneficial power of omega 3 in our diet—that's all we really need to know. We need to consume more omega 3!"

Hold the phone Lundell. If there's 4500 articles that all come to the same conclusion about the benefits of omega 3, why isn't this more publicized? Why aren't our family doctors screaming for us to change our diets?

"Sometimes even capitalism can't avoid the facts," says Lundell. "There is one clever pharmaceutical company that has now received FDA approval for an omega 3 formulation, called Omacor. Hey, I have to give them credit for promoting a healthy product. One also has to admire their ability to take something relatively inexpensive, make it a prescription drug and be able to charge a huge premium—that's good business. But, it's not really necessary when we can get the same results simply by consuming more in other natural ways. Interestingly, in Japan, omega 3 has been a prescription drug for many years and just recently it has been approved for over-the-counter use. We'll probably see the same trend here in the states. However, those of you reading this book will be far ahead of the game."

OMEGA 3 FACTS

THREE MAIN TYPES:

ALA:	Alpha-linoleic acid
Source:	From plants mostly
EPA:	Eicosapentanoic acid
Source:	From fish and marine algae

DHA:	Docosahexanoic acid
Source:	From fish and marine algae

We get enough ALA
We need more EPA and DHA

CAUTION!!!!!
*If the label does not say EPA and DHA
it is probably ALA you don't need it!*

*Use only high concentration purified fish oil
with at least 500 mg combined EPA and DHA*

HOW PURE IS YOUR OMEGA 3?
Simple test to see if you supplement is high quality: put it in the freezer for 24 hours if it turns cloudy it is not purified high quality!!

Fire Extinguisher #2—Douse the Fat?

Another essential free fatty acid that has shown major benefits in our battle is called conjugated linoleic acid or CLA.

This one, everybody will love!

"CLA cannot be synthesized in our bodies therefore we must obtain it from our diet," says Dr. Lundell. "The dietary sources of CLA are dairy products, and meat—the same foods that we haven't been eating because the establishment and public consensus have deemed them the evil foods."

CLA as a supplement was originally studied for its anticancer effects. However, further studies on animals and humans have demonstrated some interesting and potentially very exciting, beneficial effects—anti-inflammatory and weight management.

Too good to be true? Nope. CLA fights more than just one battle.

"CLA has been shown to reduce body fat mass and increase lean body mass both in animals and humans," says Lundell. "The size of fat cells have been shown to be reduced, and the number of fat cells has also been shown to be reduced."

Particularly, CLA has been shown to reduce abdominal fat, which is now considered a major risk factor for heart disease, especially in men. The reason abdominal fat is so dangerous is because it produces more of the cytokines, which begin the inflammatory process in the arteries. But, the reason you're probably getting excited right about now is because you're thinking about slimming down the pot belly.

"My clinical experience with CLA was very dramatic," says Dr. Lundell. "Typically, when a person loses weight, approximately 20% of the weight loss comes from the loss of lean body mass or muscle mass. When we did trials on CLA, none of our patients lost any muscle mass, in spite of significant fat loss. Plus, C-reactive protein levels fell relatively quickly into the normal range. The benefits of CLA are simply amazing."

He's right. And the list of benefits, from his clinical studies and the research of others, also reveals that:

- CLA is a significant antioxidant, which helps fight free radical damage.

- CLA increases energy and may suppress appetite.

- CLA has been shown to improve insulin sensitivity.

- CLA has been shown to be an anti-inflammatory—a natural Cox 2 inhibitor that may increase the synthesis of the anti-inflammatory prostaglandins.

- CLA reduces the production of cytokines.

- CLA reduces abdominal fat and preserves muscle mass.

"Most exciting to me is the fact that CLA has been shown to be anti-atherogenic," says Dr. Lundell. "I know; that's another big word. It means that it will both prevent and reduce the amount of plaque in the arteries. This evidence so far is based on animal experiments. However, it is the same animal model that is used to test every other anti-atherogenic drug, and every statin. In this animal model, plaques were reduced by more than 50% in a well-done experiment. There are some human studies on statins to reduce plaque. But, they've yielded minimal results even with high doses. And, statins are accompanied by a laundry list of bad side effects. Plus, if all this good news isn't enough, it turns out that CLA works better when there are adequate amounts of omega 3 in our system, and omega 3 works better when we have enough CLA. That's called synergy—they build on each other. Some times two plus two can equal six. The benefits of having both are extraordinary."

Extinguisher #3—Douse the Spark

Here's a little tidbit of advice that has become public consensus to which Dr. Lundell adds his adamant support—take your aspirin.

"Multiple observational and controlled studies demonstrate the benefits of aspirin in the battle against chronic low-grade inflammation," says Lundell. "One little baby aspirin (81 mg) daily has been shown to be enough for the average person."

Let's recap. Here's your Firefighting "To-Do" list so far.

First, we supplement our diet with omega 3 and CLA because our diets are generally deficient in these two essential free fatty acids. Both of these essential free fatty acids are anti-inflammatory and have multiple positive effects on cardiovascular health and our health in general. Omega 3 and CLA supplements work well for this, because our typical diet is so deficient. We can also increase our consumption of fatty fish to receive more omega 3, but supplements are the easiest and most easily managed means. Supplementation of CLA is also the most effective and efficient way to include it in our diet. Plus, we need to add one baby aspirin into our daily regime. Take it the same time every day so you don't forget.

Extinguisher # 4—Douse Your Body with Anti-oxidants

Remember when we talked about oxidation and its similarities to rust? Giving your body the anti-oxidants vitamins it needs to remain healthy is much like rust proofing your car. When facing certain damaging environmental elements, they are absolutely necessary.

"We know that one of the fundamental triggers of inflammation is the oxidation of LDL and other fats," says Dr. Lundell. "That means that we must have adequate intake of antioxidant vitamins and minerals to help extinguish the fire by stopping the oxidation of the fats and preventing the production of abnormal amounts of homocysteine. And, if we're not getting enough through our food supply, which few people actually are, we need to supplement our diets with antioxidants."

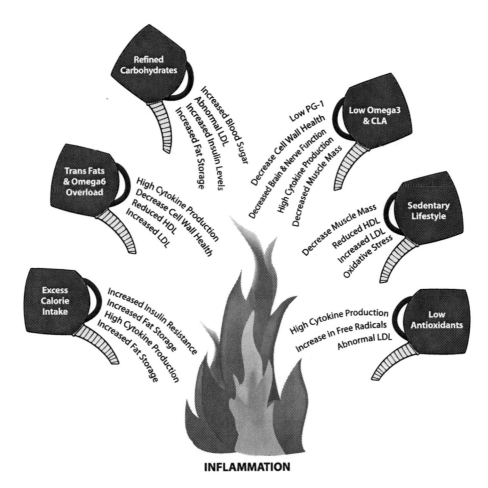

INFLAMMATION

HEART DISEASE, STROKE, DIABETES, ARTHRITIS, DEPRESSION, OBESITY, ALZHEIMER'S DISEASE, FATIGUE, LOU GERIGH'S DISEASE, LUNG DISEASE

Cool. Now we know what to add to our diet. What else do we do?

"Just like a regular fire, we started fighting with a fire extinguisher," says Dr. Lundell. "If you really want to fight this disease you've got to supplement your diet as it's nearly impossible to get the essential elements from our diet in today's world. After you supplement, or spray the extinguisher on the fire, the next thing we can do is eliminate the fuel. This is easy because we've discussed all these things already. What are the sources of fuel that cause chronic low-grade inflammation?"

Let's cut the inflammation fuel.

Fuel Source #1: Omega 6 fats—lower your consumption.

The most common sources in our diets of omega 6 essential free fatty acids are corn oil, soybean oil, safflower, and sunflower oil. In other words, all the oils we have been encouraged to eat by the "authorities" in order to avoid animal fats.

Quite simply, we need an oil change!

"The fear of fat has caused more problems than the fat itself," says Dr. Lundell. "The idea that saturated fats cause coronary disease is completely incorrect. The avoidance of animal fats and their replacement with vegetable fats plays a huge part in causing heart disease. Why is this? Because it encourages the pro-inflammatory metabolism of excess omega 6—it throws the ratio off kilter. These vegetable oils should be replaced in our diets with lard, coconut oil or olive oil."

Fuel Source #2: Hypertension—lower your blood pressure.

If you have high blood pressure, it is critical that you get treated. Everyone responds differently to anti-hypertensive medications, so consult carefully with your doctor. However, Dr. Lundell recommends a few other lifestyle changes that everyone can make to lower blood pressure. He says, "Avoid excessive salt intake. That's the first thing. Then, lose 10% of your body weight and begin to exercise. Weight loss and exercise are the most effective nonprescription methods of lowering your blood pressure. In fact, they can be much more effective than prescription medications and certainly are healthier. It has been clearly demonstrated in studies of patients who have gastric bypass surgery for morbid obesity that almost 80% are completely cured of their hypertension with weight loss. Many people struggle with weight issues. But, I'm not asking for much here—just do the math and do the exercise to lose at least 10%. It could save your life, and beyond that, I guarantee it'll make you feel a lot better about life."

He adds, "Let's not forget that each pound of fat on our body contains 3500 calories. If we reduce our food intake by only 500 calories a day, it amounts to 1 pound of weight loss per week, or 52 pounds in a year. Just skip one sweet roll per day. Or eliminate chips, snacks and sodas. Small, consistent decisions about food choices do in fact make the difference between life and death."

Mild exercise programs, such as walking or riding a bicycle for 30 minutes at least 3 or 4 times a week have proven to be extremely effective in lowering blood pressure.

If you cannot quickly get your blood pressure normal contact your doctor, get evaluated and medicated if needed. Do not delay!

"If you must be on medication, angiotensin inhibitors, or the so-called ACE (angiotensin converting enzyme) inhibitors are the best in terms of reducing inflammation in the arteries."

Fuel Source #3: Blood sugar—lower your sugar and carbohydrate consumption.

Hey, we said it before and we'll repeat it again—the most striking dietary change in the last 100 years has been the dramatic increase in our consumption of sugar. What formerly was a treat now has become a staple. Fat and protein have been replaced with simple carbohydrates—breads, cereals, and pastas. Oh yea, and all the typical American snack foods!

"Our increased consumption of sugar parallels the increase in coronary disease, diabetes and obesity," says Dr. Lundell. "This is so unbelievably obvious that it's dreadfully stupid we don't have more clarity and better advice from medical and public health authorities. We've been talking about putting out the fire of inflammation in our vessels; to continue with a high carbohydrate diet is exactly like pouring gasoline on a fire!"

Remember, every living cell in our body is interconnected. A high carbohydrate diet causes high insulin levels, which causes fat storage and inhibits fat breakdown, which leads to the production of cytokines from the overloaded fat cells, which leads to inflammation in the arteries, which leads to the devastating effects of arteriosclerosis, heart attacks, stroke, high blood pressure, kidney failure and limb loss.

Yes, that was a long-winded, run-on sentence. However, it shows just how interconnected our biological systems are in the human body. And, as much trauma that is listed in the previous paragraph that is a result of overindulging in simple carbohydrates, we're still missing one possible side effect—death.

"Our bodies aren't biologically equipped to process the agricultural, carbohydrate-heavy diet that is recommended by the government," says Dr. Lundell. "And, if we don't stop—if we don't reduce our blood sugar—the epidemic we face will continue to kill us, our children, and future generations."

Fuel Source #4: Smoking—Don't smoke 'em if you got 'em.

Let's face it, where there's smoke there's fire. The advice to avoid smoking cigarettes is so painfully obvious. It almost does not deserve discussion. However, just because there's a consensus to avoid smoking does not mean it's necessarily scientifically based. In fact, you'd think that with all the publicity surrounding the dangers of smoking that a more scientific approach would be taken.

Currently, only one third of cigarette smokers die prematurely. That's a statistic that is surprisingly low considering all the publicity the nasty habit has received. And, you could probably defend the habit by reciting the story of Uncle Joe who lived to be 90 and smoked two packs a day. Everyone has one of those stories. But, regardless of what happened to Uncle Joe, Cousin Ned, or Sister Suzy, the cigs need to be extinguished.

"Even if you've heard about the recent studies showing that nicotine by itself may be beneficial in fighting Alzheimer's, don't be fooled; this is not a plus for smoking." says Dr. Lundell. "This is one of those cases in which people need to look carefully at the research and ask some basic common sense questions. The concept that cigarette smoking causes systemic low-grade inflammation is well-documented. If something irritates our airway, our bodies have a natural reaction to the irritant—we cough. And if the irritation, from the smoke and the coughing continues, our body reacts with inflammation to defend itself. You don't need any scientific background to see how obvious it is that cigarette smoking is a cause of inflammation. And, you also don't have to be a genius to rationalize away the dangers.

Our bodies are wonderfully equipped to repair injury. One cigarette won't kill you. But why would you keep injuring yourself? Why keep pouring gas on the fire?"

Fuel Source #5: Stress—we need to chill out!

In the world that we live, it's nearly impossible to avoid stress. However, we can learn to modify our responses to stress and provide our body with the tools to reverse the negative effects.

"When we feel stressed, our adrenal glands pour out hormones to help us cope," says Dr. Lundell. "These hormones tend to constrict all our blood vessels, especially those which are not as vital to the fight or flight reaction. But, it is possible to control stress. The first step is accepting the fact that we don't always have control of our environment, but we do always have control of our reaction. Using tools like a PET scan, it has been shown that relaxation techniques can improve blood flow to the heart muscle. So, it's important that we learn how to relax. Consult with your doctor if needed. Stress is extremely dangerous. Chronic stress has been shown to increase levels of inflammatory cytokines. And, how do you feel knowing that by simply changing your reaction to stress could end the continuing battle that's waging inside your body. The brain is the powerful tool—use it."

Some common ways many people find to reduce stress are exercise, meditation, reading, or even taking a drive. Find what works for you, and make a point of finding time to relax.

Fuel Source #6: Trans-fats—eliminate them completely!

Run for your life! Run away as fast as you can! Avoid trans-fats at all costs!

"Trans-fats are poison," says Dr. Lundell. "They are. Tran-fats are similar to other fats, but they have been processed with heat and hydrogen, which changes their shape, and their function. Trans-fats are found in hydrogenated vegetable oil, partially hydrogenated vegetable oil, vegetable shortening, margarine, commercial baked goods, restaurant fried foods, cookies, crackers and chips."

Why are trans-fats so dangerous?

"They're dangerous because they interfere with the normal metabolism of omega 3. We don't get enough omega 3 to begin with, but by consuming all these trans-fats we make the deficiency even worse. Basically, trans-fats replace normal fats in the cell wall, and they interfere with the function of every cell. Remember, every cell in your body is a living, breathing thing. If we start messing with cellular function, we can quickly find ourselves in a world of pain. Consumption of trans-fats doubles the risk of heart attack."

Yikes! Double your risk of heart attack simply by consuming trans fats? That's scary.

"That's not all," says Lundell. "You don't have to die to feel the effects. Trans-fats are associated with allergic skin conditions. Trans-fats are associated with Alzheimer's disease. Trans-fats are associated with diabetes. Trans-fats are absolutely toxic."

So, is that simple or what? Scary? Maybe. But, then again, keep in mind that you're holding the fire extinguisher. You can snuff out the fire today.

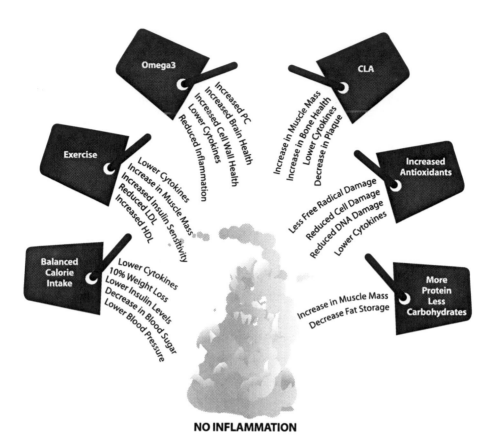

Omega3
Increased PC
Increased Brain Health
Increased Cell Wall Health
Lower Cytokines
Reduced Inflammation

CLA
Increase in Muscle Mass
Increase in Bone Health
Lower Cytokines
Decrease in Plaque

Exercise
Lower Cytokines
Increase in Muscle Mass
Reduced Insulin Sensitivity
Reduced LDL
Increased HDL

Increased Antioxidants
Less Free Radical Damage
Reduced Cell Damage
Reduced DNA Damage
Lower Cytokines

Balanced Calorie Intake
Lower Cytokines
10% Weight Loss
Lower Insulin Levels
Decrease in Blood Sugar
Lower Blood Pressure

More Protein Less Carbohydrates
Increase in Muscle Mass
Decrease Fat Storage

NO INFLAMMATION

**STABLE PLAQUE, HEALING PLAQUE, HEALTHY ARTERIES,
HEALTHY BONE & JOINTS, HEALHY BRAIN, HEALTHY BODY**

Here's the process simplified.

First, extinguish—add the proper nutrients to your diet to fight the fire. Second, cut the fuel sources—reduce, remove or eliminate the toxic substances that keep our internal blaze ignited. So far, these are easy steps. But, what about the suffocation? What about the environment that we live in today that initiates the fire—hitting us at every street corner with a fast food restaurant, bombarding us at the grocery stores with fancy and misleading packaging, and overwhelming us with stress in this rat race culture of multitasking. Reducing inflammation sounds easy on paper. What happens when you step out into the real battleground? ⊁

Living Happy and Healthy in a War Zone

IMAGINE A FIERCE BATTLEFIELD. GUNS are blazing. Bombs are exploding. People are dying. And, you're whisking gracefully through it all, whistling your favorite show tune and wondering how life could get any better.

Is it possible? Can you live healthfully and happily in a war zone?

"Am I being melodramatic, calling it a war zone?" asks Dr. Lundell. "It's ironic that many people might say that calling our current western culture a war zone might be an embellishment. But, don't forget, when you hear me say stuff like that, keep in mind that I'm a guru of the facts. 2500 people die each day of heart disease—countless more are disabled every day from heart attack, kidney failure, stroke, Alzheimer's disease, diabetes, peripheral vascular disease, and arthritis. Every single day, we see the tragic and sad casualties of war surrounding us. And, unless we are directly involved, we pretty much ignore the 2500 heart disease casualties."

Is Dr. Lundell being melodramatic? Well, no. He's not if you consider just how real those numbers are—and the families that are affected by each one of those deaths. Just imagine if another disaster killed 2500 Americans in one day. How would we respond? Can you imagine the headlines of every American newspaper? Maybe if we wrote huge, in-your-face newspaper headlines for each death or life-altering condition that was caused by chronic inflammation, the reality of our nation's health would sink in to our thick skulls. Would obnoxious headlines help the situation?

Today's Headlines Include:

Bill Jones Croaks at Age 42
Heart Attack Due to Chronic Low-Grade Inflammation Blamed

Mary Smith, Age 60—Left Leg Stolen in Amputation
Low-Grade Inflammation, Manifested as Diabetes Deemed the Thief

Tom Tomlin, Age 54, Dies of Omega 6 Overdose
Family Never Suspected Abuse— "He was a normal guy, living a typical lifestyle"

Wealthy Woman Dies of Omega 3 Starvation
Jane Jules, Age 64, Dies Painfully—Didn't Understand the Term 'Essential'

Henry Hendricks Crippled by Automobile
No Crash Involved—No Exercise Either. Henry Hasn't Taken 15 Steps Since Age 20

Misty McDaniels, Mother of 4, Poisoned by Fast Food!
Mommy-and-Me Dialysis Programs Filled—Children Fend for Themselves

Okay. So these headlines seem almost silly. But, sadly, these head-lines happen every single day. And, if we weren't all so entrenched in what the public consensus deems as acceptable and healthy, we might respond more aggressively to such tragedies.

What if, instead of Dr. Lundell saying, "2500 people die each day from heart disease," you woke up to your morning newspaper and it read:

Town of Happyville Wiped Out Overnight—2500 Dead!
Experts Blame Local Culture—"No One Can Survive the Inflammation Epidemic"

Would you want to live there? Would you think differently about the situation our nation faces?

"For some reason, we blame a lot of health issues on age," says Lundell. "The deaths, disabilities, and health problems in this war do not just involve people of advanced age. We are now raising the first generation of Americans who cannot expect to live longer than their parents. Why? With all the medical technology we have to save lives, we're still facing a generation that cannot overcome its own environment. We need to face the facts. We're dying. And, we're killing our children and grandchildren by allowing them to live under the same dietary misguidance."

That's a scary thought. At least if we're going to kill and disable ourselves, we could help stop the epidemic from being passed to our children and grandchildren. Even a recent anti-smoking campaign suggests, "If you won't quit smoking cigarettes, at least don't smoke around your kids." That campaign is inspired by the relatively recent research that reveals the negative health effects of second-hand smoke. And, it resonates with many parents.

"It's never too late to change," says Lundell. "Sometimes I hear people say that they don't want their children to follow in their footsteps. But, all they need to do is change their footsteps. Wouldn't it be great if a 60-year-old father could challenge his 30-year-old son to hike up a mountain, or run around the block, or to lose 15 pounds? Or, what if he could inspire him to walk through the war zone unscathed and unaffected—even laughing in the face of danger? A 30-year-old can change the national statistics today. A 70-year-old can change it. Everyone reading this book can save more lives than I ever could as a heart surgeon. We can start with our selves, our children, and our grandchildren. From there, all we need to do is inform the world—person by person. That sounds like a huge task. It's not. First, we lead by example—change our own thinking and the results will engage others to follow."

C'mon, Dr. Lundell, are you seriously trying to tell us that if we change, that the war zone around us, the overwhelming public consensus, and the political misguidance that directs our standard health recommendations, will suddenly change?

"Ironically, the public—you, me, our neighbors, families and friends—are the only people that have the power to change the system," confirms Lundell. "We're all more powerful than any heart surgeon or lobbyist or politician. We all hold the most powerful title of anyone. We are the almighty consumer."

That's it? Well, you gotta admit that it makes sense. Every day, we are bombarded with images and words scientifically designed to make decisions for us—so we'll purchase food and drink that will make us sick, and someone else, rich. And, as much as that sounds like some sort of deranged conspiracy theory, it's a fact. We're a capitalist country. It's our constitutional right to get rich. All we need to do is wrangle up consumers who will buy our products.

"It has been said that cigarettes are the only consumer product, which if used as instructed, is designed to kill you," says Dr. Lundell. "I think that is no longer true. A large order of fries containing a large amount of trans-fats, simple carbohydrates, and excess calories will ultimately have the same effect. We have just as much scientific evidence to prove that certain foods will kill you, as we do for cigarettes—if not more."

Are manufacturers killing us?

Wait a second. Are these companies really trying to hurt us?

The tobacco industry says, "No." They're simply meeting consumer demands. The food industry says, "No." They're just meeting consumer demands. The lobbyist representing the corn industry says, "No." He or she is just trying to protect their client. The lobbyist for the sugar industry or the high fructose corn syrup industry also says, "Not me. I'm merely trying to create a favorable regulatory atmosphere that will allow my client to sell more products." And, the vegetable oil industry and their lobbyist say their products are what the official government guidelines called for when they asked us to avoid animal fats. All of these groups are proud that their products are inexpensive, have a long shelf life, and are, in fact, demanded. They're not doing anything wrong. Consumer demands create wealth. These groups are giving us exactly what we ask them to give us.

Is it wrong simply because these products are unhealthy?

"No, it's not wrong," says Dr. Lundell. "It's capitalism. But, it doesn't mean that we, as consumers, need to continue buying this junk."

What about all the slick advertising? How can we resist? These companies work hard, studying consumer trends, so they can create effective advertising that influences public consensus and convinces us to demand their products. C'mon, there's nothing more appetizing than seeing a triple cheeseburger next to a fresh batch of salty fries and a 64-ounce soda on television. Then, when it's advertised at the price of just $3.99, what could be more appealing?

"If your health is collateral damage, well sorry," says Dr. Lundell. "No one has forced you to purchase these products. It's your choice."

That's fascinating. **Consider this: We're in the middle of war where we have the opportunity to choose *not* to be a victim.**

"It's our choice—my choice and yours," says Lundell. "The whole theme of this book has been to empower you to live healthy, happy, and disease free. Yes, the advertising is sometimes compelling. Yes, we like our food convenient, ready to eat, and inexpensive. Yes, we would rather passively ride than actively walk. We don't need to look very far to see the current state of thought in America—we're happy being passive. Recently, I was at an airport where at least 150 people were waiting for an elevator to take them up one floor, with the stairs immediately to their right. Why?"

The list of so-called unmotivated and lazy behavior, not to mention consumer trends in America, continues. In fact, if we made a complete list of our passive indulgences we would have enough content for another entire book. Think about it. Many of us will drive our cars around five or even ten minutes in the parking lot to get a space close to the door. Or, how many times have you seen two cars vying for the same parking spot when there's plenty of open space just thirty or 40 feet further from the door? Some of our neighborhoods no longer have sidewalks. All of our electronics now come

166

equipped with remote controls. Furniture is now being built to include refrigerators, so nobody ever needs to stand. Many of us have high-speed connections to the entertainment industry and the World Wide Web. We can be entertained, learn, and even work productively while being completely immobile. And today, many of our kitchens require only a refrigerator, a microwave, and a garbage can. Oh, and maybe a fantastic health insurance policy that would allow us to keep indulging—and give us further permission to take a seat and watch our nation die slowly in recliners.

That's not even the tip of the iceberg. What could be considered simple daily conveniences have now evolved into products which allow us to gain weight. Now we can purchase wedding bands and other jewelry that expands to growing body shapes.

Is this the new face of merchandise in America?

"All of these new conveniences make it seem like it's okay," says Dr. Lundell. "Soon, we won't have to lift a finger to do anything. Imagine that—an entire nation doing everything from an arm chair."

Of course, it's not the product manufacturer's fault. We're the one's to blame. We buy this stuff. We've brought these conditions on ourselves. We're passive. We're comfortable. We're lazy. And, that's not just laziness toward movement and exercise. We're too lazy to make our own decisions. We allow smooth talking advertising agencies to make our dietary choices. We instantly believe anything that sounds like it might be less work than our current lifestyle—like dietary recommendations that are made with sound scientific evidence. Without question, we listen to our doctors when they recommend that we take a statin to lower our cholesterol—even though you now know it's relatively unimportant.

Are doctors to blame?

Well, not really. Let's face it; our doctors don't have the time to have in-depth discussion about our personal health. They don't have time to make dietary and exercise recommendations. Plus, doctors don't get paid to give us correct diet and exercise instruction. But, they do get perks from pharmaceutical companies.

"Think about your last doctor visit," says Dr. Lundell. "You may have been there for an hour and a half, but how much time did you actually spend talking to your doctor? Once again, I'm not blaming the doctors. Most are really frustrated that they cannot spend the time necessary to help us live a healthier lifestyle. Your doctor can write your prescription for medication, and give you instructions on how to take the medication in less than five minutes. They have rooms full of patients to visit. They're busy. They get overwhelmed and stressed, like we all do. And, they want to create wealth for themselves, like we all do—as they should. They studied hard to become a doctor—so they could create a stable income. But, that leaves them in a frustrating position. They don't have the time, training, or incentive to give you the instruction we're giving you in this book."

Here's a challenge. Next time you visit your doctor, tell them that you want to live more like a hunter and gatherer—less manufactured foods, more vegetables, more lean meats, and less sugars and carbohydrates. Tell them you want to prevent, reduce, or even eliminate chronic inflammation. See what they say. Most will smile politely and respond with, "Fantastic!"

"Doctors would love for us to come in and tell them that we're now focusing on health instead of sickness," says Lundell. "The medical establishment, the pharmaceutical industry, and the hospital industry are all geared around sickness—not health. A hospital is not a healthcare facility; it's a sick-care facility. It's dedicated to treating sickness, and not health."

But, this can't be right. We have the best form of government in the world. We are all capitalists. We all appreciate the fact that our government gives every one of us the opportunity to become extremely wealthy. However, capitalism comes with a price tag. The gears of our government are lubricated with money. Cash makes government happen. And, because money lubricates government, it returns the favor by pumping money and opportunity back at those who have provided the lubrication.

"I was once involved with a small technology company," says Lundell. "I actually went to Washington to lobby for our product. The halls of the Rayburn Building were layered with people attempting to get the government to buy their product or to influence legislation to put their product in a favorable light. Indeed, some of these people represented organizations of the citizens and interest groups—allowing individual voices to be heard as our constitution promises. This is what representative government should be about—hearing the voices of the people. And, if my product, or any company's product or service, is superior to another, it is completely appropriate that I, or they, attempt to influence the government to use it for the good of all. That's exactly how it should be. And, it's very exciting to see firsthand how things work. My only disappointment was realizing how money was necessary in order to be heard. And, how policy was not influenced always by facts and science, but by those people or companies or organizations who had access to, and influence with the policymakers."

This makes the whole battle seem impossible. Are we helpless victims—being thrown on the inflammatory fire, and slowly cooked to death? Can we seize life (Carpe Vitra) and preserve or regain our health? What power do we have?

"Changing the world can seem frustrating," admits Lundell. "And, it's a tough battle. Changing our external environment is difficult, but we can change the internal environment very quickly by what we put in our bodies. What will you chose to consume; pure fuels or pollutants? There is one 'world' we can change overnight, without much of a fight—your world. You can make changes in your world. Slowly, we will change the world together."

Okay, we're all reading this and there's one huge obnoxious question at the top of our brain. Our grocery stores and restaurants (especially in today's marketplace overloaded with franchises) all stock and offer the same foods. What can we do as consumers to influence the food supply available to us?

Changing the Food Supply

Please, Dr. Lundell, don't tell us to write our congressman and ask them to change the food supply.

"This isn't about petitions or task forces," says Lundell. "All we need to do is stop buying the junk. That's the simple solution. Imagine for a minute, everyone in America decided not to buy Krispy Kreme® doughnuts. What would happen? The company would either immediately go out of business, or they would go crazy trying to find out how to please us so we would buy their product again. They don't want to make you sick; they just want to make money. And, many companies will find a way to make money from you—they want everyone to be their customer. It's as simple as that. You have the power. Don't write a letter to a politician. Write a letter to the company—make a complaint. They will listen. Their business depends on your actions and opinions. A dramatic example is the fact that Kraft Foods has now eliminated trans-fats from Oreo cookies in response to consumer demand. McDonald's now offers apples as a side dish to their children's meals. And, they've created salads for the adult population. Your power is in what you choose to do—how you live, what you eat, what you buy, and how much time you spend sitting still and not exercising. Live how you want to live—healthy and happy. Companies will react to your lifestyle."

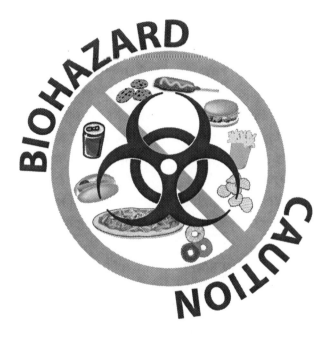

Remember, the human genome has been constant for the past 10,000 years. The only thing that has changed has been our environment. And, if you look at the past 100 years, specifically, a lot of the change has been dictated and directed by consumerism—basic supply and demand.

Yes, of course other changes have occurred in our environment, including air, water, physical activity, and our basic mode of survival.

We could certainly make the argument that our air is more polluted. However, our ancestors lived in caves huddled over smoky campfires. So, the argument may not be valid. We could also argue that our water is more polluted. And, this is true—it's disgusting how much of our water is polluted. But, at least in America, we don't drink the polluted water. Many of us even drink bottled water exclusively.

Nevertheless, with our food, dramatic changes have occurred,

Fats: Although our consumption of fat as a percentage of calories has diminished over the last 50 years, there is a dramatic shift away from animal fats and toward vegetable oil and hydrogenated vegetable oil. This has caused dangerous overdoses of omega 6 free fatty acids and artificial trans-fats. Cattle meat and dairy products—a significant source of omega 3 essential free fatty acids—no longer contain adequate amounts because livestock is grain fed instead of grass fed. Our pigs, poultry, cattle and even fish are now grain fed and therefore don't produce enough omega 3. Plus, at least for the past two or three decades, we've been discouraged from consuming any animal fat whatsoever, and encouraged to consume the vegetable oils.

Carbohydrates: Our consumption of sugar has risen from around 10 pounds per person per year in the 1890s, to about 170 pounds per person per year at present. This is because of soft drinks, added sugar to low-fat products, and our increased consumption of grains. In the last 50 years, we've increased our consumption of total grain products, from about 150 pounds per year to 200. That's nowhere near what our hunter/gatherer biology was meant to handle.

Protein: Although protein consumption in America has remained relatively constant for at least the last 50 years, its percentage of total caloric intake has dropped. Sure, we may be eating just as much protein, but it's accompanied by added calories—coming from carbohydrates and bad fats.

Hey, you don't have to be a crime scene investigator to figure out what's changed in America's diet. It's no mystery. Just poke your nose in any public garbage can—at the park or the mall or even at your office. It's loaded with soda cans, French fry wrappers, empty bags of chips, and candy bar wrappers. And, as far as activity and exercise, how many of us have gym memberships that we don't use, a dusty treadmill or piece of fitness equipment that sits idle in the corner, or an un- used pair of running shoes at the back of our closet?

All these things sound very familiar in our own lives. But, making the change seems impossible in our culture. And, if our own doctors won't or don't take the time to give us marching orders in this war zone we call life, what do we do?

Well, as luck would have it, we do have a doctor who is willing to give marching orders. What does Dr. Lundell prescribe?

Doctor's Marching Orders Through the War Zone

"Let's suppose that you (the reader) came to my office for advice on preventing coronary disease—for you and your family," says Dr. Lundell. "First we know that you and your family are living in a war zone—and have been living there for a while. Because of that, it's a safe assumption that there are at least the earliest signs of heart disease already in your arteries—they're inflamed."

"Before we get into the specifics," he says, "don't think that just because we're living in a war zone we have to live like a monk or completely isolate ourselves by hiding from everything. The old joke about the Pritikin diet was that it didn't make you live longer—it just seemed like it. In fact, my brother went to a Dean Ornish seminar several years ago, and he summarized what he learned by saying, 'If you put something in your mouth and it tastes good, spit it out! And, although both of these diet plans offer some advice that is very beneficial, they're just no fun. We can't live like that—always depriving ourselves of good tasting foods. Plus, we started this chapter by talking about living healthy and happy in a war zone. We need to give the word 'happy' just as much emphasis as the word 'healthy', or changing your lifestyle will never work."

Alright, this is progress. We can prevent heart disease, eat delicious and satisfying foods, and still enjoy life. But, what does that mean?

"If you live healthfully, life becomes much more enjoyable," says Lundell. "Most of us get fixated on how long we live. I think it's more important to focus on how healthy, and how well, we live. If you can live to the age of 90, but had two bypasses, 12 Stents, an amputation, you're blind in one eye, on dialysis, and taking $2000 worth of medication every month, do you really want to live longer? That's a horrible way to live. I've been heli-skiing with men in their late 70s. Obviously, they're still very active in their golden years. They're still mentally bright, even though some would consider heli-skiing crazy. Many are still active in businesses, professions, or volunteer activities. These people are enjoying life to its fullest. They're old men—and loving every minute!"

Almost everyone would say they want to be healthy and happy. But let's get down to some practical advice.

First:
"Grab those fire extinguishers," says Dr. Lundell. "First and foremost,

supplement your diet with omega 3. In our environment, it is diffi-cult to get enough dietary sources of omega 3. So, I strongly rec-ommend supplementing your diet with at least 3 grams of high-quality pure fish oil—high in EPA and DHA, on a daily basis. Other dietary sources of omega 3 are fatty fish—the most well-known being salmon. Have two to three servings of fish per week. Or, con-sume dietary sources like milk and eggs. Seek out the milk and eggs that come from range-fed animals if possible—they will have a higher omega 3 and lower omega 6."

Second:
"Supplement your diet with 2 to 3 grams of CLA everyday," says Lundell. "It's almost impossible to get this amount from our current dietary sources. I strongly recommend purchasing supplements with this critical free fatty acid."

Third:
"Make sure you're consuming enough vitamins and minerals," says Lundell. "In spite of our abundance of food options to provide the adequate amounts, we are still deficient in a few critical vitamins, minerals, and antioxidants. This is extremely important. Antioxidant vitamins and minerals help prevent the oxidation of lipids in our blood, which you now know is one of the initial causes of arte-riosclerosis. It's also been demonstrated that when we consume certain vitamins and minerals directly from their dietary sources like fresh fruits and vegetables, that the benefits appear to be more effective than receiving them from supplementation. However, these studies still remain inconclusive. I would always recommend eating the right foods and supplementing simply to ensure that you receive adequate amounts of necessary vitamins and minerals. I

don't, however, recommend mega doses of vitamins. But, I do recommend certain vitamin supplementation, because the evidence supports the benefit of supplementation. And, there are no side effects—there's no demonstrated harm, but there is significant potential for improved health.

What are Dr. Lundell's recommended vitamins and minerals?

- Vitamin A—5000 international units per day

- Vitamin C—500 mg daily

- Vitamin E—200 international units per day

- Vitamin B6—125 mg daily

- Vitamin B9—800 µg daily

- Vitamin B12—120 µg daily

- Selenium—70 µg daily

- Enzyme CoQ-10—30 mg daily

"All of the above should be obtained from a reputable, high-quality source," says Lundell. "Their purity is important. And, not all supplements are created equally. It's well worth it to do your research and read the labels carefully."

Fourth:
"Don't smoke cigarettes and avoid secondary smoke if possible," says Dr. Lundell. "Our lungs are wonderful organs, designed to filter

out small particles of dust and other matter that float in the air. There are small hair-like structures inside your windpipe that help propel foreign particles back up to the throat, so we can cough it out. The entire system is focused on keeping your air quality pure and healthy. Why would you want to abuse a system completely designed to purify your oxygen source by smoking two packs a day? You're shoving toxins into your lungs when they were designed to keep toxins out. Smoking is really bad news."

Fifth:

"Avoid overloading your cells with omega 6 fats. Avoid vegetable oils, margarine, foods fried in vegetable oil, and processed or pre-pared baked goods as much as possible. In fact, avoid all hydro-genated oil. Cook with butter, coconut oil, canola oil, or olive oil. It's a simple change that could save your life."

Sixth:

"Overcome your fear of fat," says Dr. Lundell. "Don't be confused here. Yes, you should be afraid of the fat around your middle—the abdominal fat and excess body fat. It's poisoning you. However, we all need to change our perspective about eating saturated animal fats. We need these fats in our diet—of course, in moderate amounts. I know many of you may still argue that fat contains 9 calories per gram of food, compared to only 4 calories per gram for carbohy-drates. But, dietary fat has been shown to slow the emptying of the stomach, slow the absorption of sugars, and provide much more sat-isfaction to hunger with a smaller amount of food. There are many fat-soluble vitamins that can only be absorbed and utilized if we have some fat in our diet. The idea here is to enjoy the taste and ensure the health benefits of good fats. Proteins and fats consumed together trigger responses in our metabolism that cause us to be satisfied with a smaller amount of food. They cause us to have a physiological response that tends to burn fat instead of store it. So, change your mind about animal fat—our ancestors never questioned it. And, they were lean and mean hunting and gathering machines."

Seventh:

"Lose 10% of your body weight," says Dr. Lundell. "High blood pressure, diabetes, and high cholesterol have all been demonstrated to be cured or dramatically improved by weight loss. And, you can achieve most of the benefits by losing as little as 10% of your body weight. I'm not asking for much here. Quite honestly, when most people see how easy it can be to lose 10%, they get inspired to continue improving their physical condition—they lose more body fat. As I mentioned before, the most damaging fat to carry around is that which is around the middle—the belly fat. Study after study has demonstrated that abdominal obesity is closely associated with a pro-inflammatory state. In two autopsy studies of young people, abdominal obesity was closely correlated to the amount of disease in their coronary arteries. We don't have to be rail thin to be healthy, but obesity is absolutely incompatible with good health. It's not about how you look. It's about the fire inside."

"Weight loss in America is a difficult proposition because of a hostile environment driven by fad diets and incomplete—and sometimes unhealthy—guidelines. But, let's be clear and simple. Losing weight isn't rocket science. It's not about the latest fad diet. In fact, it's more about the long standing history of our dietary guidelines than anything else. The magic weight loss secret is really looking back to how our ancestors lived. What has changed in our diets, causing these epidemics of coronary disease, diabetes and obesity?

178

You already know the answer to that question—and the answer is the golden key to weight loss. I can spell out why we're overweight—it's the sugar. And, it's not a new discovery. The idea that reducing our consumption of simple carbohydrates is the key to losing weight goes clear back to William Banting's letter on corpulence. The secret hasn't changed. It is not complex. All you need to do is reduce your intake of simple carbohydrates."

Ta-da! You'll magically lose weight.

"I know it's easier said than done," says Dr. Lundell. "If you keep these small tricks in mind, it'll seem like a cinch. Add more fruits and vegetables to your plate. Add more protein to your plate—especially lean cooked meats instead of fried. Remember, don't fear animal fats. The right kinds of fat and a little more protein in each meal will satisfy your hunger much longer than if you eat carbohydrates. Before long, you'll realize that you're happier, much more energetic, and quite a bit thinner.

Eighth:
"Monitor your alcohol consumption," says Dr. Lundell. "Whether you consume alcohol or not, is an individual choice. Large observational studies demonstrate a higher mortality rate in those who consume excess alcohol, and those who consume no alcohol. The lowest mortality rate is seen in moderate drinkers. Of course, there is debate as to what this means, but there is no debate about the most healthy alcoholic beverage to drink if you choose to drink—red wine. Red wine contains some interesting compounds that appear to have anti-inflammatory and anti-aging effects. Moderation is the key. And, each of us really needs to keep our drinking, if we choose to drink, in check."

Ninth:

"Get some exercise!" exclaims Dr. Lundell. "A recent study of patients with coronary disease in Europe compared the results of subjects who were given either a standard medical therapy or a bicycle. At the end of one year, the bicycle riders had a better survival rate, fewer symptoms, and a better quality of life. Exercise is key. It's critical. It's what our bodies crave for good health."

"Exercise lowers C-reactive protein, lowers inflammation, raises HDL, improves the function of blood vessels, treats anxiety and depression, builds muscle and bone, and has an enormous impact on our emotional state," he says. "Your capacity to exercise—the physical condition your body is in—is a powerful predictor of death from coronary disease. It's more accurate than measuring cholesterol levels. The best cardiologist in Arizona says, 'I can give you a bucket full of statin and lower your risk of heart attack by 30%, but if I can get you to exercise one hour a day, I'll lower your risk of heart attack by 90%.' Sure, it can be frustrating at first. It takes the average person about 40 minutes on a treadmill to burn off one chocolate chip cookie. The point is, let's not be average. Exercise is crucial in returning our human physiology to what our genome needs for healthy survival. More simply, we're genetically programmed to be active. If we're not active, were creating a physical situation that makes it difficult to adapt to our environment. A lot has been written, and there's a ton of confusion about what kind, and how much, exercise a person needs on a daily basis. I recommend we keep it simple—especially when you first start exercising. Do what you can do. Do what seems most enjoyable. Just do it. And, do it consistently. Studies show that walking 10,000 steps a day will improve your health. For many people, just taking those additional steps may be enough. However, if you're capable of doing more—and let's be honest about how much we're truly capable of doing—make it a point to make exercise happen in your life. Work up to a sweat. You're never too old. Your history doesn't matter. Exercise benefits everyone."

Dr. Lundell continues, "We all say we don't have time, but it's really the little things like taking the stairs instead of the elevator, or like parking at the far end of the lot to take a few extra steps. It's the little things like walking down the hall at work instead of picking up the phone or sending an email. Every little bit helps. And, every little bit of inactivity hurts. Get fit, bit by bit. Let me challenge everyone reading this book to ask your self one huge question. Can any of us afford not to invest at least 20 minutes a day of exercise into our schedules if it can prolong our life by decades, or make us happier and more confident people, or give us a little more energy into our golden years, or prevent illnesses that could possibly disable us from living normal lives? Hey, if you can come with me on a 50 mile bike ride that's wonderful. If you can barely make it around the block, at least it's a start. And, just so you know, I didn't start exercising until I was 40. I'm no different than you. And, today I'm riding my bike with triathletes!"

Tenth:
"Be happy," says Lundell. "Stress, which can show itself in many forms, has been shown to cause the release of cytokines—those chemicals that began the awful process of arteriosclerosis. I am not Dr. Phil, but I don't think it's too hard to figure out the things that aggravate us or make us unhappy. Change what we can, and accept what we can't. We've got one shot at this life. That alone should make each of us ask ourselves: am I living a life that makes me happy?"

Eleventh:
"Don't forget to take that baby aspirin!" says Lundell. "Aspirin,

although it seems ancient in the new world of pharmacology, is one of the most beneficial things you can do for yourself. Of course you should consult your family doctor. Please, don't let any urban myths scare you away from aspirin. Ask your doctor. For most of us, the majority of us, and almost every single one of us, aspirin is extreme ly beneficial and perfectly safe."

Twelfth:

"Write your own headline," says Dr. Lundell. "We joked about head-lines earlier in this chapter. And, I don't want to come across as some sort of motivational speaker here. However, I do want to drive home the point that to accomplish anything—with your own health, or with our nation's health—each one of us needs to step up to the plate and take ownership. I challenge each one of you to write your own headline for what you will have accomplished. Make it as off-the-wall or far-fetched as you want. But, realize after you write it, that only you have the power to make it come true—good headline or bad headline. It's your job to realize that power. Choose to live the happy and healthy life you deserve." ⟩(

ten

Homeland Security: 6 Rules of Defense

HOW MANY TIMES HAVE YOU heard statistics that flying in an airplane is safer than driving? It's true. Statistically, flying is safer. Nevertheless, millions of people are still very anxious about flying. That same irrational thought process happens every day in our lives. We'll look both ways before crossing the street to a fast food restaurant—only to poison ourselves after we cross. We buckle our children into high-tech safety seats to avoid injury, yet we drive them to the fast food place to feed them toxic food. Over time, that food will kill them. Many people will even avoid exercise by using the excuse "I don't want to over do it." Then, they under do it every night by sitting in front of the television.

Should we look both ways before crossing the street? Absolutely. Should our children be strapped in car seats? Of course they should! And, should we pay attention to our bodies to truly understand our own level of exhaustion? Yes, there's no doubt about it.

Why can't we understand that protecting our health comes in many forms? No, we don't jump out of trees to risk breaking bones. So, why do we fill ourselves with toxins to risk premature disease and death?

Let's be honest with ourselves. All of us would like to believe that we don't have any disease in our arteries. But as you learned in Chapter 1, we all have it—to some degree or another. The only question is: are you going to put out the inflammation fire to help your arteries heal, or are you going to ignore it until the plaque ruptures? Are you going to ignore your unhealthy lifestyle until you get cancer? Are you going to ignore your health until you get Alzheimer's? Are you going to ignore your health until it kills you?

Well, are you?

"The human body is incredibly resilient," says Dr. Lundell. "It can tolerate a huge amount of abuse, and still keep going. It's like a self-repairing machine. Life exposes us to insult and injury every day, but the body is built to defend, heal, and repair itself. Our cardiovascular system responds to stimuli to control our body temperature; deliver the right amount of blood to the right places, at the right time; and protect us from harm. It really is 72 miracles a minute. But, I can't stress enough the importance of self-awareness. If we inflame the lining of our blood vessels multiple times every day—by ignoring our own biological needs—the healing process can never catch up. At some point, the plaque you've built up in your artery wall will rupture and you will have a heart attack. You've read the statistics in this book. What's the greater risk of death; not buckling your seatbelt or eating super sized fries daily?"

So, how do we create a Homeland Security system for own body?

Rule #1: Prepare Your Home

"To start, we all need to fully understand that everything in our body is connected," says Dr. Lundell. "Our cardiovascular system touches and influences every single aspect of our health. Your cardiovascular system is as crucial to your health as the sun is crucial to the survival of the earth—it affects everything. To create a defense system, we start by identifying any enemies or harmful stimuli—realizing that damage to any part of your body is damage to your entire body. Then we learn to avoid any risks, and proactively learn to respond to attacks."

So, this isn't just about heart health, it's about health in general. Even gum disease is an indicator of cardiovascular illness—that's how connected the cells are within our bodies.

"Learning healthy behaviors isn't just about focusing on the heart, or the lungs, or the liver or the brain," says Dr. Lundell. "In most circumstances, if you make a healthy change to your lifestyle, it will benefit all parts of your body."

Let's start in your own home—make it an anti-inflammatory safe haven for you and your family. Go into your pantry, take a look around, and see if you have invited the enemy to live with you. Do you have chips, cookies, crackers, prepared baked goods, and vegetable oils on your shelves? Do you have instant rice, canned beans, potatoes, hydrogenated oils, candy, or enriched pasta in your cupboards? If you do, you have invited the enemy into your life.

Step 1. Get rid of the junk in your home.

"Learn to read the nutrition facts labels," says Dr. Lundell. "All foods are now required to have the nutrition facts printed clearly on their labels. It may seem confusing at first, but the more you study the nutrition facts, the easier it will become to quickly identify the foods you should not consume. Look at the carbohydrate content, the trans-fat content, and the serving size. Be aware of other parts of the label—if it says low fat, it often means high sugar. Make a plan to evict these killers from your house."

Okay, so what happens when you do a clean sweep of the cupboards, the refrigerator and the freezer into the trash? It'll seem like you have nothing to eat. And, you have to eat something. Right?

Step 2. Find replacements for the junk.
"As you clean out the cupboard, take inventory of what you're tossing so you can simultaneously make a replacement grocery list," says Dr. Lundell. "Start by replacing your vegetable oils with high-quality cold pressed or extra-virgin olive oil, grape seed or canola oil—all can be used for cooking at high temperatures. Butter should be used for baking, avocado, coconut, walnut, and hazelnut oils are good for dressing vegetables. And, olive oil and balsamic vinegar make delicious salad dressings. Replace the enemy starches with fresh fruits, fresh vegetables, and canned fruits and vegetables as long as they don't have added sugar. Frozen fruit, often has less added sugar than canned fruit."

What are the easiest things to remember when making a grocery list of healthy foods?

"First, color matters," says Dr. Lundell. "Don't eat anything white. Choose colorful vegetables, leafy vegetables, and non-starchy vegetables. Choose whole grains and cracked grains when you consume breads and pastas. But, consume in moderation. And, as difficult as it may seem, avoid refined flour products, instant rice, and potatoes. Basically, if it's white, it's not right."

When it comes to eating right, excess sugar and carbohydrates, excess hydrogenated fats (bad fats), and a deficiency of good fats will cause us to lose the battle with inflammation. However, a reduced carbohydrate diet, along with increased protein, increased omega 3, CLA, colorful vegetables and fruit, proper supplementation, and exercise will defend against inflammation. It's like creating an anti-inflammatory perimeter around your body—a strong defensive barricade against invasion.

"If you haven't done so already, go to the bookstore and get a low-carb cookbook," says Dr. Lundell. "There are many available, and most have great information. The most famous of course, are the Atkins and South Beach low-carb cookbooks."

Wait a minute. Dr. Lundell, you're not giving us the worn-out low-carb story are you? The same old weight-loss story? The trendy dieting pitch?

"No, I'm not," says Dr. Lundell. "This isn't about weight loss. This book is about inflammation. It's about having a diet that matches our genetics—so we live longer, stronger, and healthier. In fact, I'm not pitching low-carb at all. This is about normal-carb—the diet our bodies were biologically programmed to receive to naturally fight and prevent disease. It's about consuming a proper amount of carbohydrates that are high quality, contain multiple nutrients, and don't cause dangerous elevations of blood sugar and insulin. It's about a diet and lifestyle that fights inflammation instead of promoting it. Will you lose weight if you follow this diet? Yes, you will.

But, the last thing I want is for people to think that weight loss is the point. This is a healthy lifestyle, not a teeter-totter weight loss program. You will lose weight. But, more importantly, you'll lose the health risks that come from inflammation. You'll decrease your risk of disease and premature death. And, quite frankly, if you follow this plan, you'll never need to think about losing weight again—because this is a diet for life."

Want to see some differences between fad diets and lifestyle eating habits?

"Look at the comparison of the hunter/gatherer diet, with the low carbohydrate, low-fat, Mediterranean diet," says Dr. Lundell. "The key differences between these diets and the low-fat diet, are the intake of omega 3—the hunter/gatherer and Mediterranean diets both have high levels of omega 3. The fiber is also high, the amounts of fruits and vegetables are high, and the amounts of nuts and seeds are moderate. But, the refined sugars are low "

Dietary Components	Hunter–Gatherer	Mediterranean
Protein (%)	High (19 - 35)	Moderate (16 - 23)
Carbohydrates (%)	Moderate (22 - 40)	Moderate (45 - 55)
Total Fat (%)	Moderate (28 - 47)	Moderate (25 - 35)
Omega 3 intake	High	High
Fruits and Vegetables	High	High
Nuts and seeds	Moderate	Moderate
Salt	Low	Moderate
Refined Sugars	Low	Low
Glycemic load	Low	Low

We shouldn't need any more convincing about how bad the low-fat diet is for our heart and our overall health. But, what about the low-carbohydrate or zero-carbohydrate diets?

"Again, I want to stress that this isn't about weight loss," says Dr. Lundell. "And, for the most part, if some low-carbohydrate diets are actually followed properly, they can be very successful at reducing inflammation and extremely successful at losing weight. But, we're talking about curing disease. Many fruits are high in carbohydrates—and I suggest you eat them. Eat a lot of them. Several credible studies have been performed demonstrating the effects of the so-called Mediterranean diet. Really, the key benefits are the intake of omega 3 from supplements and fatty fish, as well as the intake of complex carbohydrates in the form of fruits and vegetables. Those are high carbohydrate foods. And, they'll help us live longer and stronger. Look at the dramatic Lyon Diet Heart study that compares the typical Western-style diet with the Mediterranean diet. Notice a 68% decrease in cardiac death and non-fatal heart attack. Need I say more? This isn't the same old low-carb message. It's about a balanced diet—a healthy diet. And, it's about balancing the amount of calories we consume compared to the amount of calories we burn. It's about eating good food, instead of junk food, so that we are satisfied and nourished with fewer calories."

"We are genetically programmed to be omnivores," Dr. Lundell continues. "Why fight our natural programming? Being an omnivore means we need to be eating a wide variety of foods. So, stock your cupboards with a large variety. As you read the cookbooks, you will discover an amazing variety of deliciously satisfying nutrient dense foods that will help create the perfect anti-inflammatory environment for healthy arteries. And remember, this is a war in which we can choose not to be a casualty. You fill your cupboards. You have the choice of what you put in your kitchen. And, you have the choice of what you put in your mouth."

Rule #2: Strategy for Venturing Out

Let's face reality. None of us want to live in the hunter/gatherer times. But, we might want to gather the family and hunt for a supermarket or a great restaurant. Venturing out of the safety of your own home can be scary. Most often, you're entering a danger zone filled with unhealthy temptations. Of course, this doesn't mean you can't go out on the town—dining out has become one of the most common forms of American entertainment. And, shopping—even at the grocery store—can also be considered entertainment. When you go—because you will; be prepared. Arm yourself with knowledge and a steadfast commitment to your health. When you go to the market, make it a rule to purchase the majority of your foods from the periphery aisles. In most grocery stores, the periphery or outside aisles are where you'll find the fresh fruits, vegetables, and meats. Avoid the interior aisles of the super market where they keep the processed and packaged foods like chips, crackers, cookies, and other carbohydrates like rice and pasta. Take your healthy replacement grocery list, and stick to the list. Learn to read the nutrition label. And, don't take poison back into your home.

Restaurants are another danger zone—the sights, sounds, smells, and menus are designed to entice you. Restaurants make money by selling food—so they want to serve you large portions. They want you to salivate over tastes and walk away with a savory memory. But, remember, they are concerned with your customer experience. It's your job to be concerned about your health.

"Here is a safety tip for visiting restaurants," says Dr. Lundell. "It'll sound really strange at first. But, if you practice this just a few

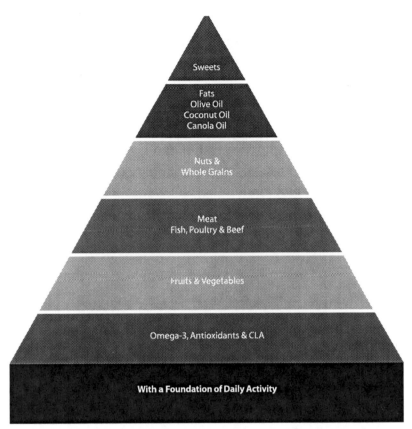

DR. LUNDELL'S I.Q. (INFLAMMATION QUOTIENT®) FOOD PYRAMID

times, you'll realize that your dining experience can even be better. If you really want to protect your health when you dine out, don't go to the restaurant hungry. Have a high-protein snack and two glasses of water before you go, and you'll tend to eat less. And, when you eat less, you'll leave that restaurant without feeling bloated, or tired, or regretful. You don't have to eat it all either. Just because the food fills the plate doesn't mean it's the proper amount to satisfy your appetite."

That might be tough for some of us. Many of us were raised in homes where you were expected to clean your plate—become a member of the "clean plate club". As children we would hear our parents say things like, "You better eat that. There are children in third-world countries who don't get anything to eat." And, even though you don't eat everything on your plate doesn't mean you can't eat all your fantastic food—it doesn't have to go to waste. Ask for a doggie bag.

"I'm not suggesting that a person can't enjoy themselves at a restaurant," says Dr. Lundell. "Have a steak, but not a potato. Dress your salad with olive oil and vinegar. Take a pass on the bread and dessert. Ask for steamed vegetable or fruit instead of pasta sides or rice. You can still enjoy your meal."

Dr. Lundell's Healthy Tips for Fast Food

Burger Chains
"Order that bacon cheeseburger," says Dr. Lundell. "Just discard the bun and avoid the ketchup and special sauce, which is very high in sugar. And, without question, leave the fries for someone else. Many burger chains now offer complete meals with options like side salads instead of fries. Use those options. And, one of the best things you can do is order water as your beverage."

Sandwich Shops
"Sandwiches may seem a lot healthier because the meats aren't fried, but that's not really what is causing the problem," says Dr. Lundell. "The same thought process for sandwich shops needs to hold true as it did for burger chains. Enjoy the meats, cheeses and vegetables—just discard the roll, bread or bun. In fact, look at the sandwich shop's salad menu. Many times you can get your favorite sandwich in a bowl. It tastes just as good and is much better for you."

Salad Bars

"Dieters love to eat at salad bars," says Dr. Lundell. "However, often people miss the healthy benefits because they assume that everything is healthy because it comes from a salad bar. Choose a base of non-starchy vegetables. Go for the green stuff and top it off with proteins such as hardboiled eggs, turkey, and chicken. Pass on the pasta salad and skip the baked potato."

Fried Chicken Shops

"Believe it or not, there is healthy food everywhere," says Dr. Lundell. "And, it tastes fantastic!" If you go to a fried chicken restaurant, avoid barbecued, breaded, and deep-fried chicken. Most stores offer grilled or roasted chicken instead. And, for the side dishes, stay away from the rolls and mashed potatoes. Ask for vegetables, fruits or even yogurt as your side dish."

Other Chains

"I understand that it's difficult to find quick, easy, and healthy choices at many of the fast food restaurants out there," says Dr. Lundell. "We have choices of Italian, Japanese, Chinese, and Mexican food chains. Plus, it seems there's a new franchise tempting your taste buds every day. The key to eating healthy at all of these restaurants is avoiding starches—skip the buns, breads, noodles and rice. Go for the vegetables and meats. And, have fun discovering new healthy options within menus."

Eating can be a challenge. But as you have learned, it is the small daily decisions that make the difference in the battle against inflammation. And, keep in mind that all the new healthy options that appear on menus all across the fast food industry were created because people like you demanded healthy options. It's really that simple. If we ask for better options, sooner or later, these restaurants will want to sell us a healthy meal.

Rule #3: Assess Your Battlefield

Is testing for arterial disease necessary?

You may have been intrigued by a lot of the information provided in this book. Hopefully, you're inspired to change your life today. However, many people reading this book will consume the information and passively slide right back into their old unhealthy habits. Maybe you'll go to the grocery store and buy some eggs with a commitment in your mind to eat more protein. Maybe you'll buy some fresh fish to help increase your omega 3 intake. And, maybe you'll run to your health food store and buy some high quality supplements. Yet, statistically, many of you will still say, "good enough" because you don't know exactly how much inflammation already exists in your body.

"Remember, I'm a guru of the facts," says Dr. Lundell. "The fact is that all of us have some damage already. The war we've been talking about is raging inside your body and creating some type of negative side effect. It is a fact. I live and breathe this information and I have inflammation. I have plaque. This is why it's important to assess yourself. If you're the type of person who needs to know how bad the damage is to motivate you into action, modern medicine has many tools to provide that assessment. And, in my opinion, anything that motivates you into living healthier is well worth investigating."

Health Screening Options:

Test your I. Q. Inflammation Quotient ™

Go to www.InflammationQuotient.org for a simple self-test to estimate your level of inflammation.

   • **Test your CRP.** "C-reactive protein is now a widely available medical test," says Dr. Lundell. "And, it will soon become widely used as an indicator for heart disease. Basically, the test measures the level of C-reactive protein in our blood. This gives us an indication of the amount of inflammation in our body. Normally there is very little C-reactive protein circulating in our blood. The lowest risk is 1.0 or below, while moderate risk is 1.0 to 3.0. And anything above 3.0 is significant risk for coronary disease and other inflammation-related disorders. The next time you have blood work done, asks your doctor to measure it. If it's elevated, you need to get serious and work really hard to get it below 1.0. The amount of C. reactive protein in your blood is as good of an indicator for coronary artery disease, or possibly better, than LDL. You may have to ask for the test now, but very soon it will become standard procedure."

   • **Test your homocysteine levels.** "Homocysteine directly damages the lining cells of the arteries and needs to be controlled," says Dr. Lundell. "High levels of homocysteine indicate low levels of critical B vitamins especially B12 and B9 (sometimes referred to as folic acid). Homocysteine levels can easily be lowered with supplements."

   • **Test your omega 3 index.** "Your omega 3 index measures the amount of omega 3 in the cell walls of your red blood cells," says

Dr. Lundell. "This is a relatively new test. However, it has been well established and documented as a powerful indicator of coronary artery disease. This test is not yet widely available, but if you'll contact me, I will personally arrange for you to have it. You can find my contact information at www.DoctorLundell.com. The great thing about this test is that if you are deficient, it has been clearly demonstrated that we can increase our omega 3 levels with supplementation and intake of appropriate fish."

• **Have a stress echo and stress nuclear scan performed.** "A stress echo test is where you walk on a treadmill and the function of your heart is assessed by ultrasound," says Dr. Lundell. "This examination is important to know whether our heart muscle is being starved for blood by a narrowed artery. Echocardiograms also demonstrate the function of the four valves in our heart. This test can also be done by injecting an isotope in the blood to demonstrate and/or expose those areas that are not getting enough blood. These tests are not routine and are usually given only if someone has a symptom that may indicate coronary disease. Nevertheless, it doesn't mean you cannot ask for the tests."

• **Get a CT or MRI scan.** Both CT scans (sometimes referred to as Cat scans) and MRI scans are getting dramatically more sophisticated. Both provide detailed information, not only about the size of the lumen on the artery, but also about the nature of the plaque. That means that scans can now tell us whether the plaque in your arteries is stable. Stable plaque means that the plaque has healed and has a nice fibrous cap. Unstable plaque means it has thin fibers and is likely to rupture, which could cause a heart attack. CT scanning can also measure the calcium in the coronary arteries. It will give you a "calcium score," which is an indication of the amount of plaque that exists in your arteries. Both tests are expensive but provide an extremely detailed picture of your coronary arteries.

• **Have carotid ultrasound performed**. Carotid ultrasound can provide extremely valuable information simply by placing the ultrasound probe on our neck to examine the carotid arteries—the arteries that carry blood to your brain. In the past, carotid ultrasound was only used if there was some symptom indicating significant disease in those arteries. Recently, however, it has been clearly demonstrated that the health of the carotid artery is a very good indicator of the health of the rest of our arteries. Now, this has been called the surrogate marker for coronary artery disease. This test has been used widely in studies attempting to demonstrate reduction of plaque by various medications, and has been established as a standard by which to measure plaque reduction. Basically, the test measures the thickness of your artery wall, and it measures the ratio of the intima to the media. Remember the intima is the very thin lining layer of the arteries. The media is the smooth muscle layer where the disease accumulates. This test can tell you if vulnerable plaque exists in your carotid arteries. If plaque exists, you are at high risk for a stroke. This test is often referred to as CIMT (carotid intimal to medial thickness).

Which tests does Dr. Lundell recommend?

"All the tests mentioned are effective in measuring certain risk factors," says Dr. Lundell. "And, as much as I'd like to tell everyone to have every test performed, I understand that it's not a realistic request—simply due to the price. So, my simple recommendation for assessing your personal battlefield, unless you have a reason to believe you're facing sudden danger, is to first take the free 'I.Q.' Inflammation Quotient® test at my web site, www.InflammationQuotient.org. Check your C-reactive protein and homocysteine. I think it's important that everyone has a good understanding of the inflammation in their body—because inflammation can cause so many diseases. Second, have a carotid ultrasound, just to be safe. And third, if you haven't yet started taking omega 3 supplements, get your omega 3 index checked. Yes, that still sounds like a lot of tests. But, the last thing I want anyone to do is walk away from this book thinking that this epidemic hasn't touched them. It's affecting all of us—even me."

Rule #4: Train for Battle

Watch out. This is the portion of the book where Dr. Lundell tells us to get off the couch and start exercising. Maybe you already take brisk walks. Maybe you're already a runner, climber, hiker, biker, dancer, skier, or martial artist. And, if you are, that's fantastic. However, statistically, many of us are simply couch potatoes.

"Our bodies need to move," says Dr. Lundell. "Remember when you were a kid and you just had to get outside and expel energy? That's the way we're always supposed to feel. Aging doesn't mean we need to stop moving. Our bodies are capable of rigorous motion into our golden years. And, the more you exercise, the more you want to exercise. If you are a couch potato, start by getting yourself a pedometer just to count your steps in a day. Try increasing your steps by 10%. Soon, you'll want to increase those steps by 20%. Start slowly and build on your fitness. Remember, I didn't start excercising until I was 40 years old. Today, I'm training with triathletes. But, it's important that you find an activity that you like to do. Start slow, and never stop. Our nation is slowly dying on couches. Don't become one of the statistics who lose their life simply because they used the excuse that they didn't have the time to exercise. If you don't exercise, you won't be given the time to live a happy and healthy life."

Rule #5: Prepare for Friendly Fire

How many times in life are we challenged by change? It never fails. Think about the times you wanted to begin a new career. Think about the times you wanted to chase your dreams. How many of those times—when you wanted to change—did a friend or family member step in to give you a pessimistic perspective on your goal? It happens, and you can expect a little "friendly fire" from your friends and loved ones when you attempt to cure heart disease.

"Whenever we start doing something different, well-meaning friends and family (often unconsciously) try to sabotage us," says Dr. Lundell. "They often think they have some knowledge that we don't. Or, they'll bring up some weird circumstance that sheds a negative light on your will to change. But, now that you have read this book, you have more knowledge than most. In fact, you probably have more knowledge than some physicians about the health of the cardiovascular system. Expect that others will try to shut down your goals of success. Fight back. Prove everyone else wrong. You have the facts. Your biology is no different than our ancestors, and if you follow the advice in the book, you will prove the naysayers wrong. It's your life and your body. In this battle, like any battle, there will be friendly fire. And, as we all know, sometimes friendly fire can be the most dangerous to your safety. But, don't let it dissuade you from winning the war."

Rule #6: Start Your Own Army

Now that you're armed with the knowledge to protect yourself, improve your health, and that of your family, it's time to expand your sphere of influence. Share your knowledge, and please, share this book.

Ask your favorite restaurants to cook with healthy fats and eliminate all trans-fats. Ask your supermarket to carry healthy foods. If they don't, shop somewhere else. Check Appendice D for a list of web resources; do your research and continue to learn the facts. This will give you a voice in the regulatory environment.

Take control of your health. Heart disease has found a cure, and it starts with you.

"I performed more than 5000 open heart surgeries," says Dr. Lundell. "Yet, those who read this book can save many, many more lives than I ever could. That's the beauty of this book. Information is more powerful than anything else. Now you, the reader, have the power to cure. The time to fight the war is now. Your head is already into the battle. Today, you can get your heart into it." ⋊

Epilogue

Death happens only once.
Good health is a continuum.

Learning and practicing what you've learned so far will pull you out of the death zone. Sharing this knowledge will make you a lifesaver.

The next stage is to maximize health, healthy aging, well-being and the enjoyment of this life in our hostile environment.

So Dr. Lundell and Todd Nordstrom are back at it again, gathering the latest scientific research, making it understandable, demonstrating how it works in everyday life with everyday people.

In their next book they will share with you, inspiring real-life stories of the transformation that occurs when people follow their science based plan.

What's the title? That's still a secret. When will it be released?

For updates and official news, log on to **www.drlundell.com**

YOU ARE GOING TO LOVE THE NEW BOOK EVEN MORE!

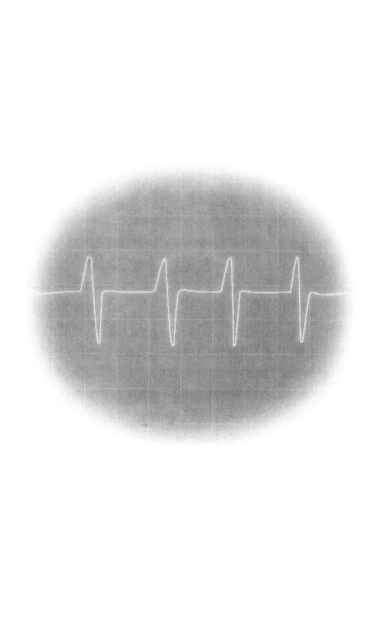

Appendices

A. Omega 3 Studies

American Journal of Clinical Nutrition
**Fish oil reduces heart disease risk in menopausal women–
Hormone Replacement Therapy or not**
Stark KD, Park EJ, Maines VA, Holub BJ. Effect of a fish-oil concentrate on serum lipids in postmenopausal women receiving and not receiving hormone replacement therapy in a placebo-controlled, double blind trial. Am J Clin Nutr 2000;72(2):389-394.

BACKGROUND: Omega-3 fatty acid supplementation lowered serum triacylglycerol concentrations in studies in which most of the subjects were male. The effects of omega-3 fatty acid supplementation in postmenopausal women receiving and not receiving hormone replacement therapy (HRT) have received little attention.

OBJECTIVE: We sought to determine the effects of a fish-oil-derived omega-3 fatty acid concentrate on serum lipid and lipoprotein risk factors for cardiovascular disease in postmenopausal women receiving and not receiving HRT, with an emphasis on serum triacylglycerol concentrations and the ratio of triacylglycerol to HDL cholesterol.

DESIGN: Postmenopausal women (n = 36) were grouped according to exogenous hormone use and were randomly allocated to receive 8 capsules/d of either placebo oil (control) or n-3 fatty acid-enriched oil (supplement). The supplement provided 2.4 g eicosapentaenoic acid (EPA) plus 1.6 g docosahexaenoic acid (DHA) daily. Serum lipids and the fatty acid composition of serum phospholipids were determined on days 0 and 28.

RESULTS: Supplementation with omega-3 fatty acids was associated with 26% lower serum triacylglycerol concentrations (P < 0.0001), a 28% lower overall ratio of serum triacylglycerol to HDL cholesterol (P < 0.01), and markedly greater EPA and DHA concentrations in serum phospholipids (P < 0.05).

CONCLUSIONS: These results show that supplementation with a fish-oil-derived concentrate can favorably influence selected cardiovascular disease risk factors, particularly by achieving marked reductions in serum triacylglycerol concentrations and triacylglycerol: HDL cholesterol in postmenopausal women receiving and not receiving HRT. This approach could potentially reduce the risk of coronary heart disease by 27% in postmenopausal women.

Annals of Internal Medicine
Fish Oils and Atherosclerosis
von Schacky, Clemens, et al. The effect of dietary omega-3 fatty acids on coronary atherosclerosis. Annals of Internal Medicine, 1999;130: 554-562.

A recent study has investigated the beneficial effects of fish oil supplementation and atherosclerosis. A randomized, double-blind, placebo-controlled clinical trial involved 162 patients with confirmed atherosclerosis. Half the patients were given 6 grams of fish oils per day for three months while the other half were given 6 grams per day of placebo capsules containing a fatty acid composition resembling that of the average European diet. After three months the dosages were reduced to 3 grams/day for a further 21 months. Angiograms were taken at the start of the trial and at the end of the two-year study period. At the end of the treatment twice as many of the patients in the fish oil group (16) showed regression of their atherosclerotic deposits when compared to the placebo group. Three patients in the placebo group suffered a non-fatal heart attack during the 2-year period as compared to only one in the fish oil group. Seven patients In the placebo group had a cardiovascular event (heart attack or stroke) as compared to only two in the fish oil group. The researchers conclude that fish oil supplementation may be beneficial for atherosclerosis patients and is safe and well-tolerated.

Annals of Internal Medicine
Results from a large, systematic review report that fish oil improves mortality, even compared to statins.
Studer M, Briel M, et al. Effect of Different Antilipidemic Agents and Diets on Mortality, A Systematic Review.   Arch Intern Med, 2005;165:725-730

BACKGROUND: Guidelines for the prevention and treatment of hyperlipidemia are often based on trials using combined clinical end points. Mortality data are the most reliable data to assess efficacy of interventions. We aimed to assess efficacy and safety of different lipid-lowering interventions based on mortality data.

METHODS: We conducted a systematic search of randomized controlled trials published up to June 2003, comparing any lipid-lowering intervention with placebo or usual diet with respect to mortality.

Outcome measures were mortality from all, cardiac, and non-cardiovascular causes.

RESULTS: A total of 97 studies met eligibility criteria, with 137,140 individuals in intervention and 138,976 individuals in control groups.

Compared with control groups, risk ratios for overall mortality were 0.87 for statins (95% confidence interval [CI], 0.81-0.94), 1.00 for fibrates (95% CI, 0.91-1.11), 0.84 for resins (95% CI, 0.66-1.08), 0.96 for niacin (95% CI, 0.86-1.08), 0.77 for n-3 fatty acids (95% CI, 0.63-0.94), and 0.97 for diet (95% CI, 0.91-1.04).

Compared with control groups, risk ratios for cardiac mortality indicated benefit from statins (0.78; 95% CI, 0.72-0.84), resins (0.70; 95% CI, 0.50-0.99) and n-3 fatty acids (0.68; 95% CI, 0.52-0.90).

Risk ratios for non-cardiovascular mortality of any intervention indicated no association when compared with control groups, with the exception of fibrates (risk ratio, 1.13; 95% CI, 1.01-1.27).

CONCLUSIONS: Statins and n-3 fatty acids are the most favorable lipid-lowering interventions with reduced risks of overall and cardiac mortality.

Any potential reduction in cardiac mortality from fibrates is offset by an increased risk of death from non-cardiovascular causes.

American Journal of Cardiology
Relationship between DHA and CRP reported

Madsen T, Skou HA, Hansen VE, et al. C-reactive protein, dietary n-3 fatty acids, and the extent of coronary artery disease. Am J Cardiol, 2001; 88(10): 1139-1142.

The acute-phase reactant C-reactive protein (CRP) has emerged as an independent risk factor for coronary artery disease. Experimental and clinical studies provide evidence of anti-inflammatory effects of n-3 polyunsaturated fatty acids (PUFA) derived from fish.

We have studied the effect of marine n-3 PUFA on CRP levels in 269 patients referred for coronary angiography because of clinical suspicion of coronary artery disease. All patients filled out a food questionnaire regarding fish intake.

The n-3 PUFA content of granulocyte membranes was determined and the concentration of CRP in serum was measured using a highly sensitive assay. The results were related to angiographic findings. CRP was significantly higher in patients with significant coronary stenoses than in those with no significant angiographic changes ($p < 0.001$), but the CRP levels were not associated with the number of diseased vessels.

Subjects with CRP levels in the lower quartile had a significantly higher content of docosahexaenoic acid (DHA) in granulocytes than subjects with CRP levels in the upper quartile ($p = 0.02$), and in a multivariate linear regression analysis, DHA was independently correlated to CRP ($R(2) = 0.179$; $p = 0.003$).

The inverse correlation between CRP and DHA may reflect an anti-inflammatory effect of DHA in patients with stable coronary artery disease and suggest a novel mechanism by which fish consumption may decrease the risk of coronary artery disease.

American Journal of Preventive Medicine
Omega-3's estimated to be more effective in preventing sudden death than automated external defibrillators (AEDs)
Kottke TE, Wu LA, Brekke LN, et al. Preventing Sudden Death with n-3 (Omega-3) Fatty Acids and Defibrillators. Am J Prev Med., 2006; 31(4): 316-323.

BACKGROUND: Because interventions that prevent and treat events due to cardiovascular disease are applied to different, but overlapping, segments of the population, it can be difficult to estimate their effectiveness if formal calculations are not available.

METHODS: Markov chain analysis, including sensitivity analysis, was used with a hypothetical population resembling that of Olmsted County, MN, aged 30 to 84 in the year 2000 to compare the estimated impact of three interventions to prevent sudden death: (1) raising blood levels of n-3 (omega-3) fatty acids, (2) distributing automated external defibrillators (AEDs), and (3) implanting cardioverter defibrillators (ICDs) in appropriate candidates. The analysis was performed in 2004, 2005, and 2006.

RESULTS: Raising median n-3 fatty acid levels would be expected to lower total mortality by 6.4% (range from sensitivity analysis=1.6% to 10.3%). Distributing AEDs would be expected to lower total mortality by 0.8% (0.2% to 1.3%), and implanting ICDs would be expected to lower total mortality by 3.3% (0.6% to 8.7%).

Three fourths of the reduction in total mortality due to n-3 fatty acid augmentation would accrue from raising n-3 fatty acid levels in the healthy population.

CONCLUSIONS: Based on central values of candidacy and efficacy, raising n-3 fatty acid levels would have about eight times the impact of distributing AEDs and two times the impact of implanting ICDs.

Raising n-3 fatty acid levels would also reduce rates of sudden death among the subpopulation that does not qualify for ICDs

Arteriosclerosis, Thrombosis, and Vascular Biology
Omega-3 Fatty Acids and Cardiovascular Disease
Kris-Etherton PM, Harris WS; Appel LJ, for the AHA Nutrition Committee. Omega-3 Fatty Acids and Cardiovascular Disease. New Recommendations From the American Heart Association. Arter,Thromb & Vasc Bio.,2003;23:151-152.

Since the original American Heart Association (AHA) Science Advisory was published in 1996, important new findings have been reported about the benefits of omega-3 fatty acids on cardiovascular disease (CVD).

Omega-3 fatty acids are obtained from two dietary sources: seafood and certain nut and plant oils. Fish and fish oils contain the 20-carbon eicosapentaenoic acid (EPA) and the 22-carbon docosahexaenoic acid (DHA), whereas canola, walnut, soybean, and flaxseed oils contain the 18-carbon alpha-linolenic acid (ALA). ALA appears to be less potent than EPA and DHA.

The evidence supporting the clinical benefits of omega-3 fatty acids derive from population studies and randomized, controlled trials, and new information has emerged regarding the mechanisms of action of these nutrients. These are outlined in a recent Scientific Statement, "Fish Consumption, Fish Oil, Omega-3 Fatty Acids and Cardiovascular Disease."

Biomedicine and Pharmacotherapy
The Importance of the Ratio of Omega-6/
Omega-3 Essential Fatty Acids
SIMOPOULOS A. *The importance of the ratio of omega-6/omega-3 essential fatty acids. Biomed Pharmacother, 2002; 56(8): 365-379*

Several sources of information suggest that human beings evolved on a diet with a ratio of omega-6 to omega-3 essential fatty acids (EFA) of approximately 1 whereas in Western diets the ratio is 15/1-16.7/1.

Western diets are deficient in omega-3 fatty acids, and have excessive amounts of omega-6 fatty acids compared with the diet on which human beings evolved and their genetic patterns were established.

Excessive amounts of omega-6 polyunsaturated fatty acids (PUFA) and a very high omega-6/omega-3 ratio, as is found in today's Western diets, promote the pathogenesis of many diseases, including cardiovascular disease, cancer, and inflammatory and autoimmune diseases, whereas increased levels of omega-3 PUFA (a low omega-6/omega-3 ratio) exert suppressive effects.

In the secondary prevention of cardiovascular disease, a ratio of 4/1 was associated with a 70% decrease in total mortality. A ratio of 2.5/1 reduced rectal cell proliferation in patients with colorectal cancer, whereas a ratio of 4/1 with the same amount of omega-3 PUFA had no effect.

The lower omega-6/omega-3 ratio in women with breast cancer was associated with decreased risk.

A ratio of 2-3/1 suppressed inflammation in patients with rheumatoid arthritis, and a ratio of 5/1 had a beneficial effect on patients with asthma, whereas a ratio of 10/1 had adverse consequences.

These studies indicate that the optimal ratio may vary with the disease under consideration. This is consistent with the fact that chronic diseases are multigenic and multifactorial.

Therefore, it is quite possible that the therapeutic dose of omega-3 fatty acids will depend on the degree of severity of disease resulting from the genetic predisposition.

A lower ratio of omega-6/omega-3 fatty acids is more desirable in reducing the risk of many of the chronic diseases of high prevalence in Western societies, as well as in the developing countries, that are being exported to the rest of the world.

Journal of the American Medical Association
Benefit vs. risk: Omega-3s significantly reduce
coronary death and mortality
Mozaffarian D, Eric B. Rimm EB. Fish Intake, Contaminants, and Human Health. Evaluating the Risks and the Benefits. J Am Medical Assoc,2006;296(15):1885-1899.

CONTEXT: Fish (finfish or shellfish) may have health benefits and also contain contaminants, resulting in confusion over the role of fish consumption in a healthy diet.

EVIDENCE ACQUISITION: We searched MEDLINE, governmental reports, and meta-analyses, supplemented by hand reviews of references and direct investigator contacts, to identify reports published through April 2006 evaluating (1) intake of fish or fish oil and cardiovascular risk, (2) effects of methylmercury and fish oil on early neurodevelopment, (3) risks of methylmercury for cardiovascular and neurologic outcomes in adults, and (4) health risks of dioxins and polychlorinated biphenyls in fish.

We concentrated on studies evaluating risk in humans, focusing on evidence, when available, from randomized trials and large prospective studies. When possible, meta-analyses were performed to characterize benefits and risks most precisely.

EVIDENCE SYNTHESIS: Modest consumption of fish (eg, 1-2 servings/wk), especially species higher in the n-3 fatty acids eicosapentaenoic acid (EPA) and docosahexaenoic acid (DHA), reduces risk of coronary death by 36% (95% confidence interval, 20%-50%; $P<.001$) and total mortality by 17% (95% confidence interval, 0%-32%; $P = .046$) and may favorably affect other clinical outcomes. Intake of 250 mg/d of EPA and DHA appears sufficient for primary prevention.

DHA appears beneficial for, and low-level methylmercury may adversely affect, early neurodevelopment. Women of childbearing age and nursing mothers should consume 2 seafood servings/wk, limiting intake of selected species.

Health effects of low-level methylmercury in adults are not clearly established; methylmercury may modestly decrease the cardiovascular benefits of fish intake. A variety of seafood should be consumed; individuals with very high consumption (5 servings/wk) should limit intake of species highest in mercury levels. Levels of dioxins and polychlorinated biphenyls in fish are low, and potential carcinogenic and other effects are outweighed by potential benefits of fish intake and should have little impact on choices or consumption of seafood (women of childbearing age should consult regional advisories for locally caught freshwater fish).

CONCLUSIONS: For major health outcomes among adults, based on both the strength of the evidence and the potential magnitudes of effect, the benefits of fish intake exceed the potential risks. For women of childbearing age, benefits of modest fish intake, excepting a few selected species, also outweigh risks.

Journal of the American Medical Association
**Consuming fish and omega-3 fatty acids from fish
reduce risk of heart disease in women**
Hu FB, Bronner L, et al. Fish and Omega-3 Fatty Acid Intake and Risk of Coronary Heart Disease in Women. JAMA. 2002;287(14):1815-1821.

CONTEXT: Higher consumption of fish and omega-3 fatty acids has been associated with a lower risk of coronary heart disease (CHD) in men, but limited data are available regarding women.

OBJECTIVE: To examine the association between fish and long-chain omega-3 fatty acid consumption and risk of CHD in women.

DESIGN, SETTING, AND PARTICIPANTS: Dietary consumption and follow-up data from 84,688 female nurses enrolled in the Nurses'

Health Study, aged 34 to 59 years and free from cardiovascular disease and cancer at baseline in 1980, were compared from validated questionnaires completed in 1980, 1984, 1986, 1990, and 1994.

MAIN OUTCOME MEASURES: Incident nonfatal myocardial infarction and CHD deaths.

RESULTS: During 16 years of follow-up, there were 1513 incident cases of CHD (484 CHD deaths and 1029 nonfatal myocardial infarctions). Compared with women who rarely ate fish (<1 per month), those with a higher intake of fish had a lower risk of CHD. After adjustment for age, smoking, and other cardiovascular risk factors, the multivariable relative risks (RRs) of CHD were 0.79 (95% confidence interval [CI], 0.64-0.97) for fish consumption 1 to 3 times per month, 0.71 (95% CI, 0.58-0.87) for once per week, 0.69 (95% CI, 0.55-0.88) for 2 to 4 times per week, and 0.66 (95% CI, 0.50-0.89) for 5 or more times per week (P for trend =.001). Similarly, women with a higher intake of omega-3 fatty acids had a lower risk of CHD, with multivariable RRs of 1.0, 0.93, 0.78, 0.68, and 0.67 (P<.001 for trend) across quintiles of intake. For fish intake and omega-3 fatty acids, the inverse association appeared to be stronger for CHD deaths (multivariate RR for fish consumption 5 times per week, 0.55 [95% CI, 0.33-0.90] for CHD deaths vs 0.73 [0.51-1.04]) than for nonfatal myocardial infarction.

CONCLUSION: Among women, higher consumption of fish and omega-3 fatty acids is associated with a lower risk of CHD, particularly CHD deaths.

Council for Responsible Nutrition News
Evidence the strongest for EPA and DHA for heart health
CRN ISSUES WHITE PAPER ON THE IMPORTANCE OF OMEGA-3 FATTY ACIDS FOR HEART HEALTH? Evidence is Strongest for EPA and DHA? Council for Responsible Nutrition

WASHINGTON, D.C., July 20, 2005

The Council for Responsible Nutrition's (CRN) Omega-3 Working Group (O3WG) today released a white paper highlighting the importance of omega-3 fatty acids, especially EPA (eicosapentaenoic acid) and DHA (docosahexaenoic acid), for heart health.

Ian Newton, executive director, CRN O3WG, stated, "As scientific research builds for the benefit for marine-based omega-3s (EPA and DHA) and consumer interest in these products continues to grow, it is important to educate various audiences on the benefits obtained from the different types of omega-3 fatty acids. The CRN O3WG white paper helps clarify some of the differences."

Two government agencies, including the Food and Drug Administration (FDA) and the Agency for Healthcare Research and Quality (AHRQ), along with the American Heart Association (AHA), have independently reviewed the available evidence and all have reached a similar conclusion: when it comes to omega-3s and heart health, the evidence is strongest for EPA and DHA.

FDA has permitted use of a qualified health claim for dietary supplements and conventional foods containing EPA and DHA, stating, "Supportive but not conclusive research shows that consumption of EPA and DHA omega-3 fatty acids may reduce the risk of coronary heart disease." This health claim does not apply to omega-3 derived from plants such as flax or canola.

AHRQ, which is part of the U.S. Department of Health and Human Services, reviewed the evidence on omega-3s and cardiovascular disease in 2004 and concluded that omega-3 fatty acids help reduce the risk of having a heart attack or dying from heart disease. AHRQ noted that "the evidence is strongest for fish or fish oil," which are the primary sources of EPA and DHA.

Another omega-3 fatty acid, alpha-linolenic acid (ALA) cannot be synthesized by the body and is therefore an essential fatty acid that must be obtained from the diet. Dietary ALA sources include grains, nuts, and plant oils such as canola and flax seed.

In the body, there is limited conversion of ALA to EPA and DHA. Therefore, to assist in maintaining a healthy heart and reducing the risk of cardiovascular disease, it is critical to obtain EPA and DHA directly from the diet, which means primarily from fatty fish (such as anchovies, sardines and salmon), from dietary supplements containing fish oils or algal oils, or from traditional foods fortified with EPA and DHA.

A number of other countries have established dietary recommendations of 0.3 to 0.5 grams per day for EPA plus DHA.

The American Heart Association and the Dietary Guidelines for Americans both recommend two meals of fatty fish per week for heart health, and this would equate to about 0.5 grams per day of EPA and DHA combined.

Since most North Americans eat very little fish and consume, on average, less than 0.1 grams of EPA and DHA per day, there is a need to take dietary supplements or foods fortified with EPA and DHA to help fill this nutritional gap.

216

A copy of the CRN O3WG white paper, titled "Omega-3 Fatty Acids in Human Health: The Role of Eicosapentaenoic, Docosahexaenoic, and Alpha-Linolenic Acids in Heart Health", is available at http://www.crnusa.org/pdfs/CRNo3wg_whitepaper.pdf.

The Council for Responsible Nutrition (CRN) is one of the dietary supplement industry's leading trade associations. The CRN Omega-3 Working Group (CRN O3WG) consists of representatives from 22 fish and algal-based omega-3 ingredient suppliers and finished product manufacturers. The CRN O3WG was formed to ensure the highest standards are available for product quality and safety from manufacturers and marketers. The group also provides scientific information about the significant health benefits of marine based omega-3 EPA and DHA to ensure greater trade and consumer confidence in these beneficial nutrients.

New England Journal of Medicine
Blood Levels of Long-Chain n-3 Fatty Acids and the Risk of Sudden Death

Albert CM, Campos H, et al. Blood levels of long-chain n-3 fatty acids and the risk of sudden death. N Eng J. Med 2002. Apr 11; 346(15):1113-1118.

BACKGROUND: Experimental data suggest that long-chain n-3 polyunsaturated fatty acids found in fish have antiarrhythmic properties, and a randomized trial suggested that dietary supplements of n-3 fatty acids may reduce the risk of sudden death among survivors of myocardial infarction. Whether long-chain n-3 fatty acids are also associated with the risk of sudden death in those without a history of cardiovascular disease is unknown.

METHODS: We conducted a prospective, nested case-control analysis among apparently healthy men who were followed for up to 17 years in the Physicians' Health Study. The fatty-acid composition of previously collected blood was analyzed by gas-liquid chromatography for 94 men in whom sudden death occurred as the first manifestation of cardiovascular disease and for 184 controls matched with them for age and smoking status.

RESULTS: Base-line blood levels of long-chain n-3 fatty acids were inversely related to the risk of sudden death both before adjustment for potential confounders (P for trend = 0.004) and after such adjustment (P for trend = 0.007). As compared with men whose blood levels of long-chain n-3 fatty acids were in the lowest quartile, the relative risk of sudden death was significantly lower among men with levels in the third quartile (adjusted relative risk, 0.28; 95 percent confidence interval, 0.09 to 0.87) and the fourth quartile (adjusted relative risk, 0.19; 95 percent confidence interval, 0.05 to 0.71).

CONCLUSIONS: The n-3 fatty acids found in fish are strongly associated with a reduced risk of sudden death among men without evidence of prior cardiovascular disease.

American Journal of Clinical Nutrition
Fish oil supplementation helps reduce inflammation, helps immune response
Trebble T, Wootton S, et al. Prostaglandin E2 production and T cell function after fish-oil supplementation: response to antioxidant co-supplementation. Am J Clin Nutr 2003;78(3):376-382

BACKGROUND: Prostaglandin E2 (PGE2) inhibits lymphocyte prolifieration and the production of interferon-gamma (IFN-gamma) by peripheral blood mononuclear cells, but the effect of PGE2 on interleukin 4 (IL-4) production is unclear.

Fish oil, which contains eicosapentaenoic and docosahexaenoic acids, inhibits production of PGE2. The effects of fish oil on lymphocyte proliferation and production of IFN-gamma and IL-4 are unclear and may be influenced by the availability of antioxidants.

OBJECTIVE: We investigated the effect of dietary fish oil with and without antioxidant cosupplementation on lymphocyte proliferation and the production of PGE2, IFN-gamma, and IL-4 by peripheral blood mononuclear cells.

DESIGN: Sixteen healthy men received dietary fish-oil supplements providing 0.3, 1, and 2 g eicosapentaenoic acid plus docosahexaenoic acid/d for 4 consecutive weeks each (total of 12 wk). All subjects were randomly assigned to daily cosupplementation with either antioxidants (200 mcg Se, 3 mg Mn, 30 mg RRR-alph-tocopheryl succinate, 90 mg ascorbic acid, 450 mcg vitamin A) or placebo.

RESULTS: Fish-oil supplementation decreased PGE2 production and increased IFN-gamma production and lymphocyte proliferation from baseline values. Cosupplementation with antioxidants did not affect cytokine production or lymphocyte proliferation.

CONCLUSION: Dietary fish oil modulates production of IFN-gamma and lymphocyte proliferation in a manner consistent with decreased production of PGE2, but this effect is not modified by antioxidant cosupplementation.

Current Atherosclerosis Reports
Omega-3s and modulation of inflammation

Mori T, Beilin L. Omega-3 fatty acids and inflammation. Curr Atheroscler Rep 2004; 6(6):461-467

Dietary omega-3 (n-3) fatty acids have a variety of anti-inflammatory and immune-modulating effects that may be of relevance to atherosclerosis and its clinical manifestations of myocardial infarction, sudden death, and stroke.

The n-3 fatty acids that appear to be most potent in this respect are the long-chain polyunsaturates derived from marine oils, namely eicosapentaenoic acid (EPA) and docosahexaenoic acid (DHA), and this review is restricted to these substances.

A variety of biologic effects of EPA and DHA have been demonstrated from feeding studies with fish or fish oil supplements in humans and animals. These include effects on triglycerides, high-density lipoprotein cholesterol, platelet function, endothelial and vascular function, blood pressure, cardiac excitability, measures of oxidative stress, pro- and anti-inflammatory cytokines, and immune function.

Epidemiologic studies provide evidence for a beneficial effect of n-3 fatty acids on manifestations of coronary heart disease and ischemic stroke, whereas randomized, controlled, clinical feeding trials support this, particularly with respect to sudden cardiac death in patients with established disease.

Clinically important anti-inflammatory effects in man are further suggested by trials demonstrating benefits of n-3 fatty acids in rheumatoid arthritis, psoriasis, asthma, and inflammatory bowel disorders.

Given the evidence relating progression of atherosclerosis to chronic inflammation, the n-3 fatty acids may play an important role via modulation of the inflammatory processes.

Journal of the American College of Nutrition
Beneficial effect of omega-3s on immune and inflammatory processes

Simopoulos A. Omega-3 fatty acids in inflammation and autoimmune diseases. J Am Coll Nutr 2002;21(6):495-505

Abstract: Among the fatty acids, it is the omega-3 polyunsaturated fatty acids (PUFA) which possess the most potent immunomodulatory activities, and among the omega-3 PUFA, those from fish oile-icosapentaenoic acid (EPA) and docosahexaenoic acid (DHA)are more biologically potent than alpha-linolenic acid (ALA).

Some of the effects of omega-3 PUFA are brought about by modulation of the amount and types of eicosanoids made, and other effects are elicited by eicosanoid-independent mechanisms, including actions upon intracellular signaling pathways, transcription factor activity and gene expression.

Animal experiments and clinical intervention studies indicate that omega-3 fatty acids have anti-inflammatory properties and, therefore, might be useful in the management of inflammatory and autoimmune diseases. Coronary heart disease, major depression, aging and cancer are characterized by an increased level of interleukin 1 (IL-1), a proinflammatory cytokine. Similarly, arthritis, Crohns disease, ulcerative colitis and lupus erythematosis are autoimmune diseases characterized by a high level of IL-1 and the proinflammatory leukotriene LTB4 produced by omega-6 fatty acids.

There have been a number of clinical trials assessing the benefits of dietary supplementation with fish oils in several inflammatory and autoimmune diseases in humans, including rheumatoid arthritis, Crohns disease, ulcerative colitis, psoriasis, lupus erythematosus, multiple sclerosis and migraine headaches.

Many of the placebo-controlled trials of fish oil in chronic inflammatory diseases reveal significant benefit, including decreased disease activity and a lowered use of anti-inflammatory drugs.

Appendices

B. CLA Studies

American Journal of Clinical Nutrition
Conjugated linoleic acid supplementation for 1 year reduces body fat mass in healthy overweight humans[1,2,3]

Jean-Michel Gaullier, Johan Halse, Kjetil Høye, Knut Kristiansen, Hans Fagertun, Hogne Vik and Ola Gudmundsen

BACKGROUND: Short-term trials showed that conjugated linoleic acid (CLA) may reduce body fat mass (BFM) and increase lean body mass (LBM), but the long-term effect of CLA was not examined.

OBJECTIVE: The objective of the study was to ascertain the 1-y effect of CLA on body composition and safety in healthy overweight adults consuming an ad libitum diet.

DESIGN: Male and female volunteers (n=180) with body mass indexes (in kg/m2) of 25–30 were included in a double-blind, placebo-controlled study. Subjects were randomly assigned to 3 groups: CLA-free fatty acid (FFA), CLA-triacylglycerol, or placebo (olive oil). Change in BFM, as measured by dual-energy X-ray absorptiometry, was the primary outcome. Secondary outcomes included the effects of CLA on LBM, adverse events, and safety variables.

RESULTS: Mean (± SD) BFM in the CLA-triacylglycerol and CLA-FFA groups was 8.7 ± 9.1% and 6.9 ± 9.1%, respectively, lower than that in the placebo group (P < 0.001). Subjects receiving CLA-FFA had 1.8 ± 4.3% greater LBM than did subjects receiving placebo (P = 0.002). These changes were not associated with diet or exercise. LDL increased in the CLA-FFA group (P= 0.008), HDL decreased in the CLA-triacylglycerol group (P=0.003), and lipoprotein(a) increased in both CLA groups (P< 0.001) compared with month 0. Fasting blood glucose concentrations remained unchanged in all 3 groups. Glycated hemoglobin rose in all groups from month 0 concentrations, but there was no significant difference between groups. Adverse events did not differ significantly between groups. Conclusion: Long-term supplementation with CLA-FFA or CLA-triacylglycerol reduces BFM in healthy overweight adults.

International Journal of Obesity
The effect of conjugated linoleic acid supplementation after weight loss on body weight regain, body composition, and resting metabolic rate in overweight subjects
M M J W Kamphuis, M P G M Lejeune, W H M Saris and M S Westerterp-Plantenga. Journal of Obesity (2003) 27, 840-847

OBJECTIVE: To study the effects of 13 weeks conjugated linoleic acid (CLA) supplementation in overweight subjects after weight loss on weight regain, body composition, resting metabolic rate, substrate oxidation, and blood plasma parameters.

DESIGN: This study had a double-blind, placebo-controlled randomized design. Subjects were first submitted to a very-low-calorie diet (VLCD 2.1 MJ/d) for 3 weeks after which they started with the 13-week intervention period. They either received 1.8 g CLA or placebo per day (low dosage, LD) or 3.6 g CLA or placebo per day (high dosage, HD).

SUBJECTS: A total of 26 men and 28 women (age 37.8±7.7 y; body mass index (BMI) 27.8±1.5 kg/m2).

MEASUREMENTS: Before VLCD (t=-3), after VLCD but before CLA or placebo intervention (t=0) and after 13-week CLA or placebo intervention (t=13), body weight, body composition (hydrodensito-metry and deuterium dilution), resting metabolic rate, substrate oxidation, physical activity, and blood plasma parameters (glucose, insulin, triacylglycerol, free fatty acids, glycerol and -hydroxy butyrate) were measured.

RESULTS: The VLCD significantly lowered body weight (6.9±1.7%), %body fat, fat mass, fat-free mass, resting metabolic rate, respiratory quotient and plasma glucose, insulin, and triacylglycerol concentrations, while free fatty acids, glycerol and -hydroxy butyrate concentrations were increased. Multiple regression analysis showed that at the end of the 13-week intervention, CLA did not affect %body weight regain (CLA LD 47.9±88.2%, CLA HD 27.4±29.8%, Placebo LD 32.0±42.8%, Placebo HD 22.5±37.9%). The regain of fat-free mass was increased by CLA (LD 6.2±3.9, HD 4.6±2.4%) compared to placebo (LD 2.8±3.2%, HD 3.4±3.6%), independent of %body weight regain and physical activity. As a consequence of an increased regain of fat-free mass by CLA, resting metabolic rate was increased by CLA (LD 12.0±11.4%, HD 13.7±14.4%) compared to placebo (LD 9.1±11.0%, HD 8.6±8.5%). Substrate oxidation and blood plasma parameters were not affected by CLA.

CONCLUSION: In conclusion, the regain of fat-free mass was favorably, dose-independently affected by a 13-week consumption of 1.8

or 3.6 g CLA/day and consequently increased the resting metabolic rate. However, it did not result in improved body weight maintenance after weight loss.

International Journal of Obesity
Conjugated linoleic acid (CLA) reduced abdominal adipose tissue in obese middle-aged men with signs of the metabolic syndrome: a randomized controlled trial
U Risérus, L Berglund and B Vessby. *International Journal of Obesity (2001) 25, 1129-1135*

BACKGROUND: Abdominal obesity is strongly related to metabolic disorders. Recent research suggests that dietary conjugated linoleic acid (CLA) reduces body fat and may improve metabolic variables in animals. The metabolic effects of CLA in abdominally obese humans have not yet been tested.

OBJECTIVE: To investigate the short-term effect of CLA on abdominal fat and cardiovascular risk factors in middle-aged men with metabolic disorders.

METHODS: Twenty-five abdominally obese men (waist-to-hip ratio (WHR), 1.05±0.05; body mass index (BMI), 32±2.7 kg/m2 (mean ± s.d.)) who were between 39 and 64-y-old participated in a double-blind randomized controlled trial for 4 weeks. Fourteen men received 4.2 g CLA/day and 10 men received a placebo. The main endpoints were differences between the two groups in sagittal abdominal diameter (SAD), serum cholesterol, low-density lipoprotein, high-density lipoprotein, triglycerides, free fatty acids, glucose and insulin.

RESULTS: At baseline, there were no significant differences between groups in anthropometric or metabolic variables. After 4 weeks there was a significant decrease in SAD (cm) in the CLA group compared to placebo (P=0.04, 95% CI; -1.12, -0.02). Other measurements of anthropometry or metabolism showed no significant differences between the groups.

CONCLUSIONS: These results indicate that CLA supplementation for 4 weeks in obese men with the metabolic syndrome may decrease abdominal fat, without concomitant effects on overall obesity or other cardiovascular risk factors. Because of the limited sample size, the effects of CLA in abdominal obesity need to be further investigated in larger trials with longer duration.

European Journal of Lipid Science and Technology
Safety of conjugated linoleic acid (CLA) in overweight or obese human volunteers
*Grethe Berven 1, Amund Bye 2, Ottar Hals 3, Henrietta Blankson 1, Hans Fagertun 4, Erling Thom 5, Jan Wadstein 6, Ola Gudmundsen 1 ***

The main objective of the study was to investigate the safety of conjugated linoleic acid (CLA) in healthy volunteers. The effect of CLA on body composition was also investigated.

The trial design was a randomized, double-blind placebo controlled study including 60 overweight or obese volunteers (body mass index (BMI) 27.5 - 39.0 kg/m2). The subjects were divided into two groups receiving 3.4 g CLA or placebo (4.5 g olive oil) daily for 12 weeks. The safety was evaluated by analysis of blood parameters and by clinical examinations at baseline and week 12. Vital signs and adverse events were registered at baseline, week 6, and week

12. Bio Impedance Assessment was applied for body composition measurements.

55 subjects completed the study. Adverse events occurred in 10% of the subjects. No difference in adverse events or other safety parameters was found between the treatment groups. Small changes in the laboratory safety data were not regarded as clinically significant. Moreover, no clinically significant changes in vital signs were observed in any of the groups.

In the CLA group, mean weight was reduced by 1.1 kg (paired t-test p = 0.005), while mean BMI was reduced by 0.4 kg/m2(p = 0.007). However, the overall treatment effect of CLA on body weight and BMI was not significant. There were no differences found between the groups with regard to efficacy parameters.

The results indicate that CLA in the given dose is a safe substance in healthy populations with regard to the safety parameters investigated.

Lipids
Conjugated linoleic acid isomer
effects in atherosclerosis: growth and regression of lesions.
Kritchevsky D, Tepper SA, Wright S, Czarnecki SK, Wilson TA, Nicolosi RJ.

Conjugated linoleic acid (CLA), a mixture of positional and geometric isomers of octadecadienoic acid, has been shown to inhibit experimentally induced atherosclerosis in rabbits and also to cause significant regression of pre-established atheromatous lesions in rabbits. The two major CLA isomers (cis9,trans11 and trans10,cis12), now available at 90% purity, have been tested individually for their anti-atherogenic or lesion regression potency. The two major isomers and the mixture were fed for 90 d to rabbits fed 0.2% cholesterol. Atherosclerosis was inhibited significantly by all three preparations. The two CLA isomers and the isomer mix were also fed (1.0%) as part of a cholesterol-free diet for 90 d to rabbits bearing atheromatous lesions produced by feeding an atherogenic diet. A fourth group was maintained on a cholesterol-free diet. On the CLA-free diet atherosclerosis was exacerbated by 35%. Reduction of severity of atheromatous lesions was observed to the same extent in all three CLA-fed groups. The average reduction of severity in the three CLA-fed groups was 26 +/- 2% compared with the first control (atherogenic diet) and 46 +/- 1% compared with the regression diet. Insofar as individual effects on atherosclerosis were concerned, there was no difference between the CLA mix and the cis9,trans11 and trans10,cis12 isomers. They inhibit atherogenesis by 50% when fed as a component of a semi-purified diet containing 0.2% cholesterol; and when fed as part of a cholesterol-free diet, they reduce established lesions by 26%. Reduction of atheromata to the observed extent by dietary means alone is noteworthy.

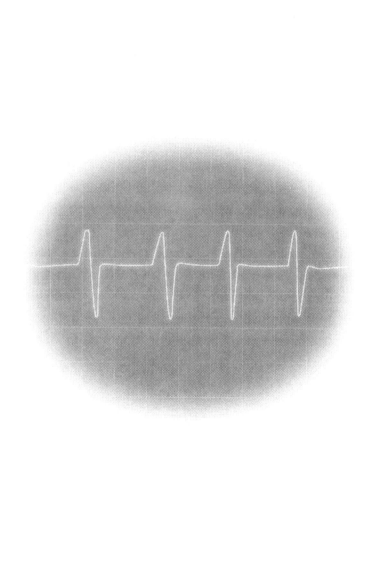

Appendices

C. ANTIOXIDANT VITAMINS
PRIMUM NON NOCERE: FIRST DO NO HARM!

This principle/precept we are all taught in medical school reminds the physician that they must consider the possible harm that any intervention might bring. It reminds us all is to examine the risk versus benefit ratio of any treatment.

The highly publicized study in the February 28, 2007 issue of the *Journal of the American Medical Association* that antioxidant vitamins increased mortality has let some physicians including the American Heart Association to advise patients not to take vitamins.

The information comes out of what is called a meta-analysis. That is to say, they took 68 studies, combine their results and did a statistical analysis. Why the vitamins were taken, the type of people who took them, sick or healthy is not analyzed. But a very, very minor increase in all-cause mortality causes "official medicine" to sound the alarm bells and frighten the 160 million people in North America and Europe, who consume vitamins.

Almost every study on statin drugs demonstrates a higher all-cause mortality when taking statins. With the benefits and only very selected groups of people. Where are the alarm bells?

They seem to have forgotten **"FIRST DO NO HARM."**

IMPORTANT FACTS:

* The best source of antioxidant vitamins is from real food.

* We don't eat enough real food and need some supplementation.

* Some of the vitamins we take routinely don't make much difference.

* Some antioxidant vitamins make a dramatic difference in human health.

* In selected groups, vitamin supplementation is critical to good health

The JAMA article and the commentators who advise against vitamins are doing more harm than good.

Appendices

D. Additional Resources

www.fatsoflife.com
This is an excellent site to learn more about Omega 3 and its health benefits. There is a newsletter and a wealth of information available here.

www.omega-research.com
An excellent, well organized site with excerpts from all the latest medical research on the health benefits of Omega 3.

www.crphealth.com
This site has all the latest research on C-reactive protein and how it affects our health. The site is sponsored by several drug companies so it's not surprising that the only treatment listed for elevated C-reactive protein is statin drugs.

www.americanheart.org
The American Heart Association is a wonderful organization and provides a wealth of information. Keep in mind that their dietary advice is incorrect!

www.InflammationQuotient.org

As mentioned, here you'll find a free and simple self-test you can use to estimate your level of inflammation. Are you at risk for heart disease? What can you do about it? Take the FREE test to find out today!

www.DoctorLundell.com

Get news and updates on cardiovascular health, comments on current health topics, access to a biweekly newsletter, diet and exercise recommendations, and a much more!

You can call 888-890-CURE (2873) or refer to the book's website www.thecureforheartdisease.net to find more detailed information on:

* Special quantity pricing for:
Non-profit Organizations
Health Care Professionals & Organizations
Corporate Wellness Programs

* Dr. Lundell is available to speak to your group or organization! Lively. Informative. Motivational. Life saving! Let your group-meet the heart surgeon who is revolutionizing the way we think about heart disease!

Printed in the United States
76841LV00002BB/121-249

9 780979 034008